Praise for *The Joy of Movement*

"In this outstanding contribution to the science of well-being, Kelly McGonigal has written a fascinating book on the complex links between physical movement, mental health, and prosocial behavior. Beautifully written and brimming with historical reflections and modern scientific findings, this is a book to savor."

—Paul Gilbert, PhD, OBE, author of *The Compassionate Mind; Mindful Compassion;* and *Overcoming Depression*

"*The Joy of Movement* will be required reading for athletes of all types, from professionals to people starting their first walking programs. Kelly McGonigal's empathy shines through the stories and research, providing a jolt of energy that will make any reader feel like the athlete they are. We aren't sure what was more fun—sitting down and reading the book, or putting it down and moving with big smiles."

—Megan Roche, MD, and David Roche, authors of *The Happy Runner*

"*The Joy of Movement* illuminates why we feel most alive when in motion, and how exercise builds social connections, both while we're working out and during the many hours a day we're not."

—Scott Douglas, author of *Running Is My Therapy*

the JOY of MOVEMENT

HOW EXERCISE HELPS US FIND

happiness,

hope,

connection,

and courage

KELLY McGONIGAL, PhD

AVERY | AN IMPRINT OF PENGUIN RANDOM HOUSE | NEW YORK

AVERY

AN IMPRINT OF PENGUIN RANDOM HOUSE LLC
penguinrandomhouse.com

First trade paperback edition, 2021

Most Avery books are available at special quantity discounts for bulk purchase for sales promotions, premiums, fund-raising, and educational needs. Special books or book excerpts also can be created to fit specific needs. For details, write SpecialMarkets@penguinrandomhouse.com.

ISBN 9780525534105 (hardcover)
ISBN 9780525534112 (ebook)
ISBN 9780593087442 (export edition)
ISBN 9780525534129 (paperback)

Printed in the United States of America
ScoutAutomatedPrintCode

Book design by Lorie Pagnozzi

To all the movement instructors who have inspired me,
and to all those who have moved with me in classes
over the years, thank you for sharing the joy.

CONTENTS

INTRODUCTION

There are very few memories I can look back on and say with certainty, "That was a moment my life changed." One of them took place when I was twenty-two. I was a graduate student in psychology and enrolled in a seminar called The Psychology of Shyness. I had always been a shy kid, and I continued to struggle with anxiety. Our project for the course was to take action on something that was important to us but that we had avoided out of fear or self-doubt. I chose to pursue my life-long dream of becoming a group exercise instructor. I had grown up doing workout videos in my living room. While other kids fantasized about becoming the next Sally Ride or Steven Spielberg, I imagined myself leading a room full of people in step-touches and jumping jacks. In high school, I studied both Spanish and French because I had read that you needed to speak three languages to teach aerobics at a Club Med resort.

Now I found myself standing outside an exercise studio on campus, minutes away from auditioning to teach for the aerobics program. Despite having practiced for so many hours that I could perform the choreography in my sleep, familiar sensations of panic flooded my system. I felt sick to my stomach. My fingernails dug into my palms. This mattered so much to me, I thought my heart was going to burst. I was overcome by the desire to rescue myself from my escalating anxiety. To just walk away, go back to my apartment, and pretend the whole thing never happened.

I remember this moment clearly, standing outside the studio, wanting to run—but choosing to stay. Maybe you've had a moment like this, too—a turning point where you said yes to something that you both dreamed about and were terrified by. Looking back, I think one of the reasons I stayed was everything I had learned about courage from my favorite forms of exercise. From yoga, I had learned how to take a deep breath and stretch beyond my comfort zone. From dance, I had learned that no matter how worried and discouraged I felt at the beginning of class, the music and movement would transport me to a state of optimism. And from my toughest cardio workouts, I had learned that a pounding heart is not always a sign of fear. Sometimes, it is proof that your heart is being strengthened.

The decision to stay and audition changed my life because it set me on the path of teaching group exercise. In the nearly two decades since, teaching has become a source of tremendous joy and meaning. Over the years, I saw again and again how movement could shift a person's mood. How it could send someone back into the world renewed with hope. I got to witness how exercise could empower participants to sense their own strength, or give them permission to let loose. As I taught individuals of all ages and varied physical abilities, I learned how movement could serve so many roles. It was a way to practice self-care, an opportunity to tackle challenges, and a place to make friends.

Many of the classes I taught turned into communities that not only moved together, but also supported and celebrated one another. In these classes, I learned what collective joy feels like, in both the synchrony of our steps and in the group hugs when a participant returned after a long absence. Leading group exercise was so fulfilling that I never stopped. It wasn't just the satisfaction of sharing the joy of movement that kept me going; it was also how movement helped me. Exercise has, at various times in my life, rescued me from isolation and despair, fostered courage and hope, reminded me how to experience joy, and given me a place to belong.

Mine is not an uncommon story. Around the world, people who are physically active are happier and more satisfied with their lives. This is true whether their preferred activity is walking, running, swimming, dancing, biking, playing sports, lifting weights, or practicing yoga. People who are regularly active have a stronger sense of purpose, and they experience more gratitude, love, and hope. They feel more connected to their communities, and are less likely to suffer from loneliness or become depressed. These benefits are seen throughout the lifespan. They apply to every socioeconomic strata and appear to be culturally universal. Importantly, the psychological and social benefits of physical activity do not depend on any particular physical ability or health status. They have been demonstrated in people with chronic pain, physical disabilities, serious mental and physical illnesses, and even among patients in hospice care. The joys described above—from hope and meaning to belonging—are linked first and foremost to *movement*, not to fitness.

The question of how physical activity contributes to human happiness is the central focus of this book. I started by scouring the science, skipping the countless surveys that show that people who exercise are happier, and searching instead for studies and theories that could shed light on why. I pored through academic papers in fields as wide-ranging as neuroscience, paleontology, and musicology. I talked to anthropologists, psychologists, and physiologists. I interviewed athletes and exercise professionals. I visited places where people move together—gyms, dance studios, parks, even an aircraft carrier. I devoured memoirs and studied ethnographies to better understand the role that movement has played across cultures and history. I expanded my search to include the writings of philosophers and religious scholars. I downloaded podcasts and joined groups on social media. I reached out to friends, family, and strangers, and asked them to share their experiences of movement. After nearly every one of these interviews, I found myself relistening to some part of the recorded conversation. Not just to check my notes, but because I wanted to hear their stories again. Many of the individuals I spoke with were brought to tears as they explained what movement meant to them. By the third time I found myself typing, "She teared up while telling me about this," I realized: These were tears of joy, and the joy of movement is moving.

One of the first things I discovered is that the most common explanation for why exercise makes us happy is far too simplistic. The psychological effects of movement cannot be reduced to an endorphin rush. Physical activity influences many other brain chemicals, including those that give you energy, alleviate worry, and help you bond with others. It reduces inflammation in the brain, which over time can protect against depression, anxiety, and loneliness. Regular exercise also remodels the physical structure of your brain to make you more receptive to joy and social connection. These neurological changes rival those observed in the most cutting-edge treatments for both depression and addiction. The mind-altering effects of exercise are even embedded in your musculature. During physical activity, muscles secrete hormones into your bloodstream that make your brain more resilient to stress. Scientists call them "hope molecules."

Looking at the evidence, it's hard not to conclude that our entire physiology was engineered to reward us for moving. But why would human biology be so finely tuned to encourage us to be active? A reasonable first guess might have to do with the health benefits of exercise. Perhaps the brain is looking out for the body, making sure we stay active enough to ward off a heart attack. Yet this notion takes too brief a historical perspective on the value of physical activity to human survival. Your doctor might encourage you to exercise to better control your blood sugar, lower your blood pressure, or reduce your risk of cancer. But for most of human existence, the central purpose of movement was not to prevent disease. Physical activity was how we engaged with life. As neuroscientist Daniel Wolpert writes, "The entire purpose of the human brain is to produce movement. Movement is the only way we have of interacting with the world." This is why our biology includes so many ways to reward moving. At the most fundamental level, rewarding movement is how your brain and body encourage you to participate in life. If you are willing to move, your muscles will give you hope. Your brain will orchestrate pleasure. And your entire physiology will adjust to help you find the energy, purpose, and courage you need to keep going.

There is also a more complex story to tell about why movement is rewarding—one that emerges from the psychology of human happiness. Human beings are hardwired to take pleasure in the activities, experiences, and mental states that help us survive. This goes beyond the obvious practical matters, such as eating and sleeping, to include many of the psychological traits that define us as humans. We enjoy cooperating and find teamwork fulfilling. We delight in making progress and take pride in what we contribute. We form attachments to people, places, and communities, and we experience a warm glow when we care for them. Even our ability to find meaning in life is rooted in the neurobiology of pleasure: stories and metaphors captivate the brain's reward system, encouraging us to craft narratives that help us make sense of our lives. Human beings do not need to re-create these habits of happiness with each new generation. These instincts are buried in our DNA and spring to life in each of us, as fundamental to our survival as the abilities to breathe, digest food, and pump blood to our muscles.

Physical activity—whether through exercise, exploration, competition, or celebration—makes us happier because it stimulates these instincts. Movement is intertwined with some of the most basic human joys, including self-expression, social connection, and mastery. When we are active, we access innate pleasures, from the satisfaction of synchronizing to the beat of music to the sensory thrill of moving with speed, grace, or power. Movement can also fulfill core human needs, such as the desires to connect with nature or to feel a part of something bigger than yourself. The physical pastimes we are most drawn to seem uniquely devised to harness our individual strengths—the abilities to persist, endure, learn, and grow—while simultaneously rousing our instincts to work together. When physical activity is most psychologically fulfilling, it's because our participation both reveals the good in us and lets us witness the good in others. This is one reason every culture puts movement at the heart of its most joyous and meaningful traditions. As philosopher Doug Anderson observed, "Movement has the power to bring us fully to what is most human about us."

As I investigated the many links between movement and happiness, this book became, by necessity, an exploration of what is most human about us. It is the only way to understand the joys of movement. And perhaps more than anything else, what I was reminded of is that human happiness flourishes in community. Human beings evolved as social creatures, and we need one another to survive. Throughout human history, movement—whether labor, ritual, or play—has helped us to connect, collaborate, and celebrate. Today, physical activity continues to draw us together and remind us how much we need one another. This was something of a revelation—how much the individual psychological benefits of physical activity rely on our social nature. How so much of the joy of movement is actually the joy of connection.

When I started writing this book, I thought it would be a self-help guide, explaining how to find happiness through exercise. It turned out to be something bigger: a love letter to movement in all its forms and also to human nature. In some strange and wonderful way, working on this book has had the same elevating effect on me as movement itself. It has given me a feeling of hope and fellowship. More than once after I finished talking to someone for the project, I said out loud, "I love humans. People are incredible." I think this was something my heart needed as much as it needs any cardiovascular exercise. Maybe it's something you need, too. If so, I hope that reading this book will give you a bit of what writing it has provided me. I hope that this book will encourage you to rethink why movement matters. I hope it will inspire you to move in ways that bring you joy and meaning. And I hope that at some point you will put this book down with a heart that is full. That you will find yourself thinking, *How marvelous, how miraculous, we humans can be.*

Chapter 1

THE PERSISTENCE HIGH

The runner's high is often held up as a lure for reluctant exercisers, described in terms that strain credulity. In 1855, Scottish philosopher Alexander Bain described the pleasure of a fast walk or run as "a species of mechanical intoxication" that produces an exhilaration akin to the ancient ecstatic worship of Bacchus, the Roman god of wine. In his memoir *Footnotes*, cultural historian Vybarr Cregan-Reid also likens his highs to inebriation. "They are as strong as bootleg whisky. They make you want to stop everyone that you pass and tell them how beautiful they are, what a wonderful world this is, isn't it great to be alive?" Trail runner and triathlete Scott Dunlap sums up his running high this way: "I would equate it to two Red Bulls and vodka, three ibuprofen, plus a $50 winning Lotto ticket in your pocket."

While many runners favor comparisons to intoxicants, others liken the high to a spiritual experience. In *The Runner's High*, Dan Sturn describes tears streaming down his face during mile seven of his morning jog. "I flew closer and closer to the place mystics and shamans and acidheads all try to describe. Each moment became precious. I felt simultaneously all alone and completely connected." Still others draw parallels not to alcohol or religion, but to love. On a Reddit forum dedicated to explaining what the runner's high feels like, one user posted, "I love what I'm doing and love everyone I see." Another offered, "It's like when you fancy someone and they tell you that they like you too." Ultrarunner Stephanie Case describes her midrun glow this way: "I feel connected to the people around me, the loved ones in my life, and I'm infinitely positive about the future."

While runners have a reputation for praising the exercise high, the side effect is not exclusive to running. A similar bliss can be found in any sustained physical activity, whether that's hiking, swimming, cycling, dancing, or yoga. However, the high emerges only after a significant effort. It seems to be the brain's way of rewarding you for working hard. Why does such a reward exist? And more important, why would it make you feel *loving*?

The latest theory about the runner's high makes a bold claim: Our ability to experience exercise-induced euphoria is linked to our earliest ancestors' lives as hunters, scavengers, and foragers. As biologist Dennis Bramble and paleoanthropologist Daniel Lieberman write, "Today, endurance running is primarily a form of exercise and recreation, but its roots may be as ancient as the origin of the human genus." The neurochemical state that makes running gratifying may have originally served as a reward to keep early humans hunting and gathering. What we call the runner's high may even have encouraged our ancestors to cooperate and share the spoils of a hunt.

In our evolutionary past, humans may have survived in part

because physical activity was pleasurable. In our modern landscape, that same high—whether you achieve it through running or some other physical activity—can elevate your mood and make social connection easier. Understanding the science behind the runner's high can help you capitalize on these effects, whether your goal is to feel more connected to your community or to find a form of exercise that leaves you love-drunk and glad to be alive.

• • •

In 2010, anthropologist Herman Pontzer was startled awake in his nylon tent by the sound of lions roaring. Pontzer, who is now a professor at Duke University, was camped near Lake Eyasi in northern Tanzania. The campsite was not far from the Olduvai Gorge, where one of the first hominid species to use tools, *Homo habilis*, lived two million years ago. Ponzter was in Tanzania to observe the physical activity habits of the Hadza, one of the last hunter-gatherer tribes in Africa. He and his team had only been at the Hadza campsite for a couple of days, and Pontzer was still getting used to the environment. He estimated that the roaring lions were no more than half a mile away. Pontzer tried to push the sounds out of mind and went back to sleep.

The next morning, he woke at six and joined his research team around a fire. As they boiled water for instant coffee and oatmeal, a group of Hadza men walked into camp carrying huge pieces of a hooved animal over their shoulders. These men had heard the same lions that had woken Pontzer, but instead of going back to sleep, they had left camp in the dark, tracked the lions, and taken their prey, a practice known as meat pirating. "Nothing makes you feel less adequate as a man," Pontzer recalls, "than sitting there eating your bowl of instant oatmeal while five Hadza guys come back with a freshly killed antelope that they stole from a pride of lions."

This stark difference between Hadza and Western lifestyles was exactly what Pontzer and his colleagues were in Tanzania to study. The Hadza live in an environment close to the one in which modern humans evolved, and analyses of their DNA reveal that they are one of the oldest human lineages on earth. The Hadza are by no means walking fossils. They are as evolved as any human being you'd find anywhere on the planet. However, their culture has not changed at the same rapid rate as those of other societies. For the three hundred or so Hadza who still follow a hunter-gatherer lifestyle, their survival depends on strategies similar to those that early humans relied on. As one of Pontzer's colleagues told me, if you want to understand what human life was like in the distant past, "This is as close as you can get." And if you want to understand the type of physical activity that the human body and brain are adapted for, this is your best chance to see it in action.

The Hadza spend most of the day hunting and foraging. Men head out in the early morning, carrying handmade bows and poison-tipped arrows to stalk everything from small birds to baboons. (The first time Pontzer went on a hunt with two Hadza men, they tracked the blood trail of a single wounded warthog for hours.) Women spend the morning collecting berries and baobab fruit and digging starchy tubers out of the ground. They carry up to twenty pounds of food back to camp, then go out again in the afternoon. As part of Pontzer's research project, his team gave nineteen Hadza men and twenty-seven Hadza women activity trackers and heart rate monitors, then recorded their dawn-to-dusk activity. On a typical day, the Hadza engage in two hours of moderate to vigorous activity, like running, and several more hours of light activity, like walking. There is no difference in activity level between men and women or between young and old. If anything, the Hadza become more active as they age. Contrast this to the United States, where the average adult engages in less than ten minutes of moderate to vigorous activity a day, and physical activity peaks at age six. If the Hadza lifestyle reflects what human bodies are adapted for, something has gone seriously awry for the rest of us.

It's worth noting that the Hadza show no signs of the cardio-vascular disease so prevalent in industrialized societies. Compared to age-matched Americans, the Hadza have lower blood pressure and healthier levels of cholesterol, triglycerides, and C-reactive protein, a measure of inflammation in the blood-stream that predicts future heart attacks. These signs of heart health are exactly what you'd expect to see in a population with high levels of physical activity. But Pontzer told me that he was even more personally struck by the apparent absence of two other modern epidemics among the Hadza: anxiety and depression. Whether this has anything to do with their active lifestyle is impossible to say, but hard not to speculate about. In the United States, daily physical activity—as captured by an accelerometer—is correlated with a sense of purpose in life. Real-time tracking also shows that people are happier during moments when they are physically active than when they are sedentary. And on days when people are more active than their usual, they report greater satisfaction with their lives.

Other experiments in the U.S. and the UK have forced moderately active adults to become sedentary for a period of time, only to watch their well-being wither. Regular exercisers who replace physical activity with a sedentary activity for two weeks become more anxious, tired, and hostile. When adults are randomly assigned to reduce their daily step count, 88 percent become more depressed. Within one week of becoming more sedentary, they report a 31 percent decline in life satisfaction. The average daily step count required to induce feelings of anxiety and depression and decrease satisfaction with life is 5,649. The typical American takes 4,774 steps per day. Across the globe, the average is 4,961.

Humans weren't always hunters and foragers. Two million years ago, a major climactic event cooled the Earth and changed the landscape of East Africa. Forested areas became more patchy and transformed into open woodlands and grasslands. As the habitat changed, so did the food supply, forcing early humans to travel far and wide to chase animals, scavenge for carcasses, and gather plants. Anthropologists believe this was a turning point in the evolution of our species—the moment natural selection began to favor physical traits that helped our ancestors run. The humans who survived were the ones whose bodies could endure the hunt.

Running doesn't fossilize, but skeletons do, and the human fossil record clearly shows the appearance, over the past two million years, of anatomical adaptations that make running possible. Predecessors to modern humans were walking upright over four million years ago, but those hominins—who spent some of their time in trees—didn't have the right feet for running. Theirs were flexible and curved, with long toes suited for clasping branches. Feet more like ours, stiffer and non-grasping, and better able to push off the earth, first show up in fossils dated to between one and two million years ago. This is around the time period you also start to see *Homo erectus* skeletons with thighbones 50 percent longer than earlier hominids, as well as wider shoulders and smaller forearms—all changes to the human form that support a more efficient running stride.

Leave the fossil record aside and you can observe many features in your own physique that help you run. Large gluteal muscles and longer Achilles tendons propel us forward. Compared to other primates, humans have more slow-twitch muscle fibers, which resist fatigue, and more mitochondria in running muscles, allowing them to consume more oxygen as fuel. We are also the only primate to have a nuchal ligament, the strip of connective tissue that fixes the base of the skull to the spine. This ligament—shared by other running species, such as wolves and horses—keeps your head from bobbing when you run. All of these adaptations suggest that we evolved as endurance athletes. Because the survival of early humans depended on traveling far and fast, you were born with bones, muscles, and joints that help you go the distance.

David Raichlen, an anthropologist at the University of Arizona, was familiar with the idea that natural selection favored traits that allowed humans to run. His own work in graduate school helped establish the theory, including a 2005 academic paper titled, "Why Is the Human Gluteus So Maximus?" But he was stymied by the problem of motivation. Nature can build a skeleton that makes running easier, but that alone is not enough to create an endurance athlete. What would make early humans willing to exert so much effort? If anything, humans seem predisposed to conserve energy. It's a caloric risk to travel all day, using up your energy reserves in the hopes of catching something big. As Herman Pontzer puts it, hunting and gathering is "a high-stakes game in which the currency is calories and going bust means death." Hunting and gathering all day can also be painful, tiring, and boring. Was an empty stomach sufficient to make a person persist on an all-day hunt or put up with the demands of foraging from dawn to dusk?

Raichlen is a recreational runner, and he began to think about the runner's high. No one had ever come up with a good explanation for why it exists. What if the high wasn't some random physiological by-product of running long distances, but nature's reward for persisting? Was it possible that evolution had found a way to harness the brain's feel-good chemicals to make endurance exercise rewarding? Maybe, Raichlen mused, early humans got high when they ran so that they wouldn't starve. He reasoned that such a neuro-reward would have to do two things: relieve pain and induce pleasure. Scientists have long speculated that endorphins are behind the runner's high, and studies show that high-intensity exercise causes an endorphin rush. But Raichlen had in mind another candidate, a class of brain chemicals called endocannabinoids. These are the same chemicals mimicked by cannabis, or marijuana. Endocannabinoids alleviate pain and boost mood, which fit Raichlen's requirements for rewarding physical labor. And many of the effects of cannabis are consistent with descriptions of exercise-induced highs, including the sudden disappearance of worries or stress, a reduction in pain, the slowing of time, and a heightening of the senses.

Earlier research had hinted that exercise might trigger a release of these brain chemicals, but no one had ever documented it during running. So Raichlen put regular runners through treadmill workouts of differing intensities. Before and after each run, he drew blood to measure endocannabinoid levels.

Walking slowly for thirty minutes had no effect. Nor did the most intense workout, running at maximum effort. Jogging, however, tripled the runners' levels of endocannabinoids. Moreover, the elevation in endocannabinoids correlated with the runners' self-reported high. Raichlen's hunch was correct. The runner's high is a buzz.

Why did jogging increase endocannabinoids, but walking slowly and running at an exhausting pace did not? Raichlen speculates that our brains reward us for exercising at intensities similar to those successfully used for hunting and foraging two million years ago. If that is true, then natural selection should also have rewarded other animals who hunt or scavenge in similar ways. Canines, for example, evolved to chase prey over large distances. Raichlen decided to put pet dogs on his treadmill, too, to see if they got a high. (Wolves would have made even better candidates for the study, but it's easier to get dogs to cooperate.) As a comparison group, Raichlen recruited pet ferrets. Wild ferrets are nocturnal, hunting small mammals asleep in their burrows. They also forage for toads, bird eggs, and other food sources unlikely or unable to lead the ferrets in a wearying chase. Natural selection had no reason to reward ferrets for physical endurance—and apparently it didn't. After thirty minutes of jogging, the dogs showed increased blood levels of endocannabinoids. The ferrets, despite trotting on the treadmill at an impressive speed of 1.9 miles per hour, did not.

What does all this mean for today's recreational exerciser? For one thing, it suggests that the key to unlocking the runner's high is not the physical action of running itself, but its continuous moderate intensity. And in fact scientists have documented a similar increase in endocannabinoids from cycling, walking on a treadmill at an incline, and outdoor hiking. If you want the high, you just have to put in the time and effort. Consider Julia, who was diagnosed twenty-two years ago with a rare genetic form of spinocerebellar ataxia, a progressive disease with symptoms that include balance problems, tremors, and muscle spasms. Julia is retired and lives alone, and one of the most important things in her life is maintaining the mobility she needs to babysit her grandchildren. So every morning she walks 500 meters (about a third of a mile) and climbs 140 stairs in her apartment building. Her family helped her calculate the distance and put together a playlist for her to listen to when she trains. The other residents in her building support Julia when they see her out; they refer warmly to her as being "on patrol." These daily sessions challenge Julia enough to give her a high. As she explains it, "I must be getting a kick from it because I really enjoy it. . . . Is it adrenaline you get when you—the walkers, the marathon runners—I think I might be getting a bit of, is it heroin?"

Anything that keeps you moving and increases your heart rate is enough to trigger nature's reward for not giving up. There's no objective measure of performance you must achieve, no pace or distance you need to reach, that determines whether you experience an exercise-induced euphoria. You just have to do something that is moderately difficult for you and stick with it for at least twenty minutes. That's because the runner's high isn't a *running* high. It's a *persistence* high.

If you were to see Jody Bender, a thirty-year-old human resources manager, on one of her frequent runs through her neighborhood park in Austin, Texas, one of the first things you might notice is her right leg. Unlike her left leg, it's covered in tattoos. Across the front of her thigh, a black and white Pegasus stretches its wings. From her ankle to her knee, a muscular blue goat with curved horns and a golden mane stands in a field of red poppies. A lucky rabbit's foot is inked near her right foot. The lopsided distribution of tattoos is not a coincidence. When Bender was twenty-three, a stroke left her unable to feel her right leg. She was at home, trying to relieve a sore neck with a heating pad, when she was overcome by the oddest sensation—like a snake was wriggling through the left side of her skull. When she stood up, she realized she couldn't walk straight. It felt like she was on a sinking ship. She made it to the bathroom, became violently ill, crawled back to bed, and passed out.

Bender now knows that the snakelike sensation in her skull was blood seeping through her brain. She has a genetic condition, fibromuscular dysplasia, that leads to abnormally weak and easily damaged blood vessels. When she was stretching her neck, she ruptured an artery, causing a hemorrhagic stroke. In an MRI image taken one week later, you can see a white spot the size of a golf ball on the left side of her brain where blood had pooled. After the stroke, Bender was unable to feel her right leg and foot—it was if they had permanently fallen asleep. Her doctors were not sure if she would ever regain sensation. A year later, she was able to walk, but she would often trip and fall. She was on blood thinners to reduce the risk of a future stroke, and these drugs made any accident more risky. If she injured herself, her body would be unable to control the blood loss. She remembers tripping and falling outside her apartment one day while walking her dog. Lying on the sidewalk, her palm and knee bleeding from where she had broken her fall, Bender became determined to increase her steadiness and strength.

She started more intensive physical therapy, even though her doctors weren't sure it would help. In her first session, the physical therapist put her on a balance machine painted to look like a mountain range. As the platform she stood on rotated, Bender immediately fell off. Her physical therapist, a marathon runner, thought running on a treadmill would be good for developing her equilibrium. "I was like, 'Are you crazy? I'm going to fall on my face,'" Bender recalls. But her physical therapist stood by her side so Bender couldn't fall, and encouraged her to alternate walking and running for thirty seconds at a time. "It was hardly running, it was like a quick walking." It took a month of physical therapy sessions to build up to running a mile. After two months, her physical therapist challenged her to run a 5K on the treadmill. In a photo from that session, Bender is smiling, her gaze straight ahead, her therapist cheering her on. "I was so surprised I could do it," she told me. "I didn't think I would ever get to that point."

Before her stroke, Bender was decidedly not a runner. "I hated running. I don't know if I had ever run a mile in my life. If I had to run for my life, I was probably in trouble." Now she runs almost every day. She often takes her dog, Cujo, with her. ("He's the sweetest dog," Bender, who is a big horror movie fan, told me when I did at double take at the name. "He's an excellent runner. He pushes me to run faster.") She has a closet full of running shoes, and when she gets ready to go for a run, she always puts her left sock and shoe on first. She slides the left sock on by feel, then carefully tugs her right sock on by sight, trying to mimic how the left sock fits. She repeats this with her sneakers. The routine takes several minutes. It's the only way she can tell if her right sock and shoe are on correctly. "The lack of feeling led me to get more blisters because I simply didn't notice that side. I've run for miles with rocks in my right shoe, only to notice when I see blood on my feet afterwards."

Sometimes when she's running, Bender finds herself reflecting on her journey. "It's usually at the end of a long run. I start thinking about where I was and where I came from," she says. "Sometimes I cry when I run. I assume no one's noticing because I'm super sweaty. I'm never really sure if it's a runner's high or I just can't believe I'm able to do this. I'm so proud of myself. There was a time I couldn't, and it wasn't that long ago." The park Bender runs in has a dirt path through the woods and a creek that is difficult to cross. The terrain is irregular, with rocks that are easy to stumble on and the occasional snake to avoid. "At some point along my run, I stop looking at the ground in front of me. I stop looking for uneven trail, acorns on the path, or a curb on the street. I start looking ahead, much farther ahead. I pick up my feet. I gain the confidence to hop over the uneven trail or jump off the curb. And that's usually where the sweet spot for me is."

In the documentary *The Great Dance: A Hunter's Story*, filmmakers captured a modern-day persistence hunt. A hunter named Karoha Langwane pursues an antelope for hours across the Kalahari Desert in 120-degree heat. Craig Foster, one of the film's directors, expected that viewers would be disturbed by the scene where the antelope, chased to exhaustion, collapses in front of the hunter, who then drives his spear into the animal's chest. But filmgoers were deeply moved by the scene and by the relief on Karoha's face as his pursuit ends with the joy of knowing that he can feed his family and his tribe. As Foster told a reporter for ESPN, "People were overcome because they were seeing a deep, important part of themselves that they never knew existed."

Witnessing this aspect of our human inheritance—the ability to persist so we can survive—can be an awe-inspiring experience. But it's also something many runners and athletes glimpse directly when they choose to push past the inertia that makes it difficult to begin or the fatigue that tempts them to stop. Jody Bender told me about a recent hiking trip she and her husband had taken in Big Bend National Park in Texas. For three days, they carried the weight of their packs on their backs and covered fifteen miles through the mountains—something that would have seemed impossible back when Bender was in physical therapy, struggling to stay vertical on the balance machine painted to look like a mountain range. On that hiking trip, Bender fell a couple of times. "I was hot and I was uncomfortable, and everything hurt. I almost ran out of water," she recalls. "But the second you finish, you don't even really remember the uncomfortable parts. You remember that feeling at the end: Wow, I said I was going to do it, and it was hard, but I didn't give up, and I did it, and that's awesome."

Persistence is key to experiencing a high while exercising, but maybe that's not the best way to think about it. We don't persist so we can get some neurochemical reward; the high is built into our biology so that we can persist. Natural selection has endowed us with a way to chase our goals and keep going even when it's hard. The runner's high is the temporary reward that carries us to our bigger goals. For many, the experience of persevering is part of what gives movement meaning and what makes the experience rewarding. This is the less heralded but perhaps most lasting side effect of the persistence high: You get to experience yourself as someone who digs in and keeps going when things get tough. This is how Jody Bender sees herself now, seven years after her stroke. She attributes much of the confidence she's developed since then to running. "I know who I am," she told me. "I don't know that I did before."

• • •

Neuroscientists describe endocannabinoids as the "don't worry, be happy" chemical, which gives us our first clue about what exactly an exercise high does to your brain. Areas of the brain that regulate the stress response, including the amygdala and prefrontal cortex, are rich in receptors for endocannabinoids. When endocannabinoid molecules lock into these receptors, they reduce anxiety and induce a state of contentment. Endocannabinoids also increase dopamine in the brain's reward system, which further fuels feelings of optimism. As runner Adharanand Finn observes, "It may only be chemicals shooting around in your brain, but after a long run everything seems right in the world."

Another way to understand what endocannabinoids do is to look at what happens when you inhibit them. The now-banned weight-loss drug Rimonabant blocks endocannabinoid receptors, an effective way to suppress appetite. In clinical trials, the drug led to alarming increases in anxiety and depression, as well as four suicides. The adverse effects on mood were so pervasive and severe that the drug was withdrawn from the European market and never approved in the United States. In a potentially unwise experiment, *Vice* reporter Hamilton Morris got his hands on Rimonabant to find out what the opposite of a cannabis high feels like. As Morris describes the effects of a sixty-milligram dose, "I have never felt so un-high in my life." He is plagued by anxiety and nausea and finds himself on the verge of tears for no apparent reason. When Morris's experiment ends, his recovery could be mistaken for a runner's high. "The neurochemical floodgates have opened and there is unimaginable rebound euphoria," Morris writes. "All night I walk down the street, peaceful and optimistic, ready to high-five strangers."

Rimonabant can still be procured for scientific research, and if you give the drug to rodents who love to run, it dramatically decreases their wheel-running. (One such experiment gave some of the mice THC, the psychoactive ingredient of cannabis, instead of Rimonabant. THC didn't have any effect on how much they ran, but it's always possible it led to some interesting experiences on the wheel.) Blocking endocannabinoids also eliminates two benefits of the runner's high: less anxiety and higher pain tolerance. Mice typically fear a new environment, but after running on a wheel, they are considerably braver when placed in an unfamiliar dark box. They also show less physical discomfort—jumping and licking their hind paws—when put on a hot plate. If mice are injected with a Rimonabant-like drug before they run, they don't get these benefits. Instead, they act just as scared and hurt as mice who hadn't exercised.

These findings provide further evidence that endocannabinoids make running rewarding. They also raise intriguing possibilities about the psychological effects of our own daily workouts. It's easy to notice and savor the peak high, but we might not recognize how its underlying brain chemistry is preparing us for what comes next. The National Study of Daily Experiences tracked the physical activity and moods of over two thousand adults in the United States, age thirty-three to eighty-four, for eight days. Every night they called participants and asked them about the most stressful events of that day. On days when people were active, stressful events—such as conflict at work or taking care of a sick child—took less of a toll on their mental well-being.

In laboratory experiments, exercise can even make you immune to the panic attacks typically induced by CCK-4, a drug that triggers severe anxiety and physical symptoms like a racing heart and breathlessness. The effect of exercising for thirty minutes before being exposed to CCK-4 is equivalent to taking a benzodiazepine like Ativan, but without the sedating side effects. Think about that: Physical activity can counteract anxiety that has literally been injected into your bloodstream. I am not a morning person, but I have learned to drag myself out from under the covers, stumble to the kitchen for coffee, and exercise before I do anything else. For me, it's a survival strategy. I want to face the day as the version of myself who takes over by the time I'm done with my workout: braver, more optimistic, and ready to face whatever challenges await me.

Niki Flemmer, a thirty-seven-year-old nurse practitioner in Seattle, had gotten into a rut running a 5K on the treadmill at her gym every day. She was sick of doing the same workout by herself all the time when she heard about a local studio that offered group treadmill and rowing classes. "It sounded hard, and I didn't know if I could keep up with the intensity," she remembers. But she was also at a time in her life when she was committed to doing things that scared her, so she decided to check the studio out.

During class, everyone works at a pace that is challenging for them. One person might be running a seven-minute mile while another walks a fifteen-minute mile. Flemmer was delighted to find that in the group setting, the same physical movement means something different than it does when she exercises alone. It feels like everyone in the class is pursuing a collective goal, putting in the effort not just for themselves but also to support one another. One of her favorite parts of the workout is when the coach calls for an all-out attack, and she looks at the person on the treadmill next to her and says, "Let's kill it!" "When I see twelve people giving it their all, I often am so moved, I get tears in my eyes."

The studio is lined with mirrors, and during a recent workout, Flemmer made eye contact with a man on the treadmill behind her. "We had that moment of absolute connection, with gestures to indicate we were cheering each other on. I felt grateful. Grateful for him and his ability to show up for himself, and grateful for the human capacity to connect." This feeling lingers after class ends. "I feel more brave out in public, to make eye contact and engage people more," she told me. "It's helping me realize that everyone wants connection. Even though they might not admit it, people like it when you smile at them."

Social confidence may seem like a surprising side effect of breaking a sweat, but the chemistry of a runner's high primes us to connect. In a 2017 review of how the endocannabinoid system works in the brain, scientists identified three things that reliably amp it up: cannabis intoxication, exercise, and social connection. The three psychological states most strongly linked to low levels of endocannabinoids? Cannabis withdrawal, anxiety, and loneliness. Endocannabinoids aren't just about not worrying and being happy; they are also about feeling close to others. Higher levels of these brain chemicals increase the pleasure you derive from being around other people. They also reduce the social anxiety that can get in the way of connecting. And just as inhibiting endocannabinoids eliminates the runner's high, it also takes away the desire or ability to connect with others. Giving rats an endocannabinoid blocker makes them less interested in socializing with other rats. In mice, it makes new mothers neglect their pups.

A runner's high does the opposite: It helps us bond. Many people have told me that they use running as an opportunity to connect with friends or loved ones. John Cary, a forty-one-year-old writer and father of two, fondly remembers taking his young daughter on runs. He would put her car seat in a jogging stroller and push her up the hills and along the outdoor trails of their hometown of Oakland, California. Sometimes they practiced making animal sounds, and other times he told her about all the people in the world who loved her. "Over the course of a run, I'm able to name fifty or sixty people in her life. Whether or not she's processing it is another question, but I just love those times we have together."

I've also heard from many people who rely on a daily workout to be more caring parents or partners. After exercising, they return to their families refreshed and ready to connect. As one runner notes, "My family will sometimes send me out running, as they know that I will come back a much better person." One study found that on days when people exercise, they report more positive interactions with friends and family. Among married couples, when spouses exercise together, both partners report more closeness later that day, including feeling loved and supported.

When I came across the research linking endocannabinoids

with social connection, I thought about something else anthropologist Herman Pontzer had told me about how early humans adapted to a changing landscape. He's convinced that running is not the only factor that helped them survive. "If you had to pick one behavior that marks the beginning of hunting and gathering, that is the game changer," he said. "It's sharing."

Hunting and gathering, both as it's done among the Hadza today and as we imagine it was done hundreds of thousands of years ago, is a division of labor. Some members of the group go out hunting, while others do the more reliable work of foraging for plants. "You bring those together at the end of the day, and you share, and everyone has enough to eat," Pontzer said. Groups who were better at sharing were more likely to survive, and natural selection started favoring not just traits that enhance physical endurance, like longer leg bones, but also traits that encourage within-group cooperation. That's why humans have such big whites of the eyes; it helps us communicate through eye contact.

Another such adaptation is a neurobiological reward for sharing and cooperating, one that looks an awful lot like the runner's high. Mutual cooperation activates brain regions linked to reward, releasing a feel-good chemical cocktail of dopamine, endorphins, and endocannabinoids. Call it a cooperation high: It feels good to work with others toward a shared goal. Brain-imaging studies show that when you see the face of someone with whom you previously cooperated, it reactivates your reward system. From an evolutionary point of view, this is the neurobiological foundation of trust. It's also a kind of anticipatory high. No doubt this is part of why Niki Flemmer experiences so much joy in her group running and rowing classes. Her brain's reward system kicks in as soon as she steps into the gym and sees the face of someone she high-fived or cheered on in a previous workout.

Sharing may also be a pleasure that that draws people to exercise in groups. A woman who practices jiujitsu told me that one of her favorite parts of training is the tradition of sharing gear. "Jiujitsu gyms are like a family, and shared gear is important. It's how you're welcomed." Her first gi, the heavy cotton jacket that practitioners wear, was borrowed from a friend. Her mouth guard was a gift from another student at the gym. Taking what is offered is part of how you belong. "It's okay if you don't have something yet," she said. That gives others a chance to let you know, "We're here for you."

Evenings in Hadzaland are spent around campfires. It's a time to unwind after a day of risk-taking hunts and focused foraging. Scientists will tell you that sitting around a fire encourages social bonding. The warmth, the flickering flames, and the crackling sounds lull us into a state more receptive to the pleasures of connecting with others. As I thought about the Hadza's evening rituals, I began to wonder: What if the runner's high does something similar? Could the afterglow of physical activity make you feel more warm and fuzzy about the people you share your life with? And make coming together at the end of the day, to share stories and a meal, even more satisfying?

It seemed to me that a runner's high fueled by endocannabinoids wouldn't just make hunting and foraging more enjoyable. By priming you to connect, the high should also make sharing the spoils with your tribe more rewarding. An experiment at the Sapienza University of Rome suggests that physical activity can have this effect. Participants played an economic game that required contributing money to a communal pool. The more they contributed, the more all parties would benefit. Participants who exercised for thirty minutes before playing the game shared more than when they played the same game without exercising first.

I ran my hypothesis—that the runner's high encourages cooperation and bonding—by anthropologist David Raichlen. He thought it was plausible that exercise-induced endocannabinoids contribute to social cohesion. In fact, he had been itching to run a study looking at whether exercising with others would lead to a bigger increase in endocannabinoids than exercising alone. But I was even more interested in another possibility— that being physically active can enhance the cooperation high and help us extract even more joy from working as a team or helping others. As it turns out, I wasn't the first to consider this proposition. When you bring together the runner's high and the helper's high, the rewards go beyond a more satisfying workout. Runners become family, communities get cared for, and humans find their tribe.

• • •

Nykolette Wallace, a thirty-five-year-old administrator for the National Health Service, was running through the streets of Southeast London in a torrential downpour. Heavy rain hadn't been expected until later that evening, and she was not dressed for the weather. Her hoodie and baseball cap were inadequate defense against the deluge, and soon she was soaked. Wallace was running with a pack of volunteers for GoodGym, a London-based organization that combines running and community projects. The group was running through Wallace's own neighborhood of Lewisham to the Goldsmiths Community Centre, which provides locals with preschool, prayer groups, ballroom dance classes, chicken lunches with bingo, and sobriety support. On the way to the center, the group ran right by Wallace's home, and she was tempted to abandon the pack, dry off, and get warm. But there was so much camaraderie, she didn't want to leave. "Humans, we moan a lot: 'It's raining, I want to get inside.' We were all out there, everyone still laughing and chatting," she remembers. "We were going to do something good because we all wanted to. Nothing else mattered."

The founder of GoodGym, Ivo Gormley, used to watch exercisers running to nowhere on treadmills in gyms, and think, *What a waste of energy.* He wondered if there was a way to harness that energy. As a first experiment, Gormley sent volunteer runners to visit socially isolated older adults in London. According to government data, half the older adults in the UK say that television and pets are their only companions, and many leave the house less than once a week. Two hundred thousand older adults in England and Wales have not spoken with a friend or family member in more than a month. As one person who requested visits from a GoodGym volunteer explained, "It would be very nice to see another human being. My only friends are people on the telly." The older adults who receive visits are given the title of "coach." Their role is to keep the runners motivated by giving them somewhere and someone to run to. The runners make regular social calls to their coaches and, when needed, help out around the house with things like changing lightbulbs. Over time, these visits turn into real friendships. More than once, when a coach has fallen ill, GoodGym runners have been their only visitors in the hospital—and at discharge, they are often the ones who take the coaches back home. Sometimes the tables are turned, and it's the coach who shows up to support a GoodGym runner.

As GoodGym grew, the organization expanded its reach, connecting runners with other volunteers in their neighborhoods and sending them to all sorts of projects in their communities. Every group run starts with a warm-up, where they learn more about that day's mission. Then they run for a mile or two to the project location, maintaining a pace that lets them talk and share stories. A designated backmarker trails the pack to make sure no one gets left behind. GoodGym has also added walking groups, for those who need or prefer a slower pace. Once on site, they might sort donations, pull weeds, organize the neighborhood toy library, or, as one recent group did, cook spaghetti Bolognese and prepare beds for locals who are homeless. The day Wallace's local group got soaked in the rain en route to the Goldsmiths Community Centre, the volunteers sanded down doors and frames to prepare them for fresh paint. Busy scrubbing wood with sandpaper, Wallace forgot her cold, damp clothes and soggy sneakers. When the rain let up, the runners distributed flyers around the neighborhood for the center's upcoming Christmas Fair, where locals could enjoy mulled wine and mince pie and do some holiday shopping. After their return trek, the GoodGym volunteers cooled down with a stretch and made plans for their own Christmas get-together at a neighborhood pub.

Before GoodGym, Wallace ran for fitness only once every couple of months. Now she runs weekly with her group. "Every time I go to catch a train, I can see something I did," Wallace says. One of her favorite group tasks was planting tulips, daffodils, and pansies in new flowerpots outside the neighborhood's main shopping center. When she visited her grandmother soon after, her grandmother asked, "Did you see those giant plant pots at the Lewisham shopping center?" Wallace also has a coach in the neighborhood, a seventy-five-year-old man who lives alone. On her first visit, she was nervous, wondering, *What if he doesn't like me? What if we have nothing to talk about?* She anticipated spending fifteen minutes, but ended up staying an hour, talking about life, books, martial arts movies, and the *Blue Planet* documentary series. "I didn't think we'd have so much in common," she told me. "One day I said to him, 'I'm really happy we get on,' and he said the same thing."

Wallace is surprised by how strong her bonds have become with her local running group. She calls them her GoodGym family. When Wallace first heard about GoodGym, she was at a point in her life where she felt stuck in her daily routine. A single mom to a teenage daughter, she didn't have many friends outside her coworkers, and she longed for a greater sense of community. On the one-year anniversary of her first run with GoodGym, she got emotional just thinking about how much her fellow runners had come to mean to her. "I know I could go to these people for anything," she told me. "I've never really had that." One of Wallace's fellow Lewisham runners says that the original mission of the organization may have been to end social isolation in the elderly, but many of the volunteers feel just as isolated before they join. GoodGym has become a way to turn strangers who happen to live near one another into a tight-knit community.

Recently, GoodGym Hounslow runner Remy Maisel, who was recovering from strep throat, tweeted, "Tonight @goodgym came to MY rescue! I'm home sick, and was really sad to be missing my group run, until @GGHounslow came to me with my favourite treats to get through another day of bedrest. Thanks, guys." The accompanying photo showed crispy mac 'n' cheese bites, a white chocolate raspberry muffin, and a get-well card. Her tweet reminded me that sharing food is such a deep and primal part of how we know we belong to a tribe. Her tribe was making sure she was fed. How strange and lovely that the evolution of the runner's high might have something to do with this part of human nature. How marvelous it is that by exercising or volunteering in packs, we can forge friendships that nourish us.

REFLECTING ON THE RUNNER'S HIGH, ultra-distance runner Amit Sheth wrote, "Helen Keller said, 'The best and the most beautiful things in the world cannot be seen or even touched. They must be felt with the heart.' The experience of bliss while running is one of them." When I read this, I thought he could just as easily have been describing the joy of belonging.

It's a puzzling marriage, running and belonging. Why do our brains so readily link physical activity and social connection? And why does the biology of the runner's high coincide so closely with the neurochemistry of cooperation? Whatever the reason, this is how we evolved. We are able to persist, for ourselves and for one another. Whether chasing down dinner, pushing a stroller up a hill, or running errands for a neighbor, we can take joy in the effort. And the more physically active you are, the more rewarding these experiences become. That's because one of the ways that regular exercise changes your brain is by increasing the density of binding sites for endocannabinoids. Your brain becomes more sensitive to any pleasure that activates the endocannabinoid system; it can take in more joy. This includes the runner's high, which helps explain why people find exercise more enjoyable the more they do it. But it also includes social pleasures, like sharing, cooperating, playing, and bonding. In this way, regular exercise may lower your threshold for feeling connected to others—allowing for more spontaneous feelings of closeness, companionship, and belonging, whether with family, friends, or strangers.

At first glance, the runner's high seems an unlikely antidote to social isolation. And yet the neurobiological reward that kept our ancestors from starving may now save us from a more pressing hunger in modern society—loneliness. The link between physical activity and social connection offers a compelling reason to be active. It also serves as an important reminder that we humans need one another to thrive.

Chapter 2

GETTING HOOKED

I n the late 1960s, Brooklyn-based psychiatrist Frederick Baekeland was trying to recruit exercisers for a sleep study. His last
experiment had shown that exercise helps people sleep more
soundly, and he wanted to test whether ceasing exercise would
interfere with deep sleep. All he needed was to find regular exercisers who were willing to stop for thirty days. The problem
was, nobody would sign up for the study.

Baekeland tried offering more money—significantly more
than he had paid participants in the past. As he later wrote,
"Many prospective subjects, especially those who exercised
daily, asserted that they would not stop exercising for any
amount of money." Those who were eventually enticed to enroll
complained not only of worse sleep but also of serious psychological distress induced by what they viewed as exercise deprivation.

This study, published in 1970, is widely considered the first
scientific report of exercise dependence. Since then, numerous
studies have shown that for regular exercisers, missing a single

workout can lead to anxiety and irritability. Three days without exercise induces symptoms of depression, and one week of abstinence can produce severe mood disturbances and insomnia. Hungarian exercise scientist Attila Szabo declared longer experiments in exercise deprivation "hopeless." Even if you could recruit participants, he argued, dedicated exercisers would, like addicts, cheat and lie about it.

Addiction is a popular analogy among both exercise enthusiasts and researchers. This analogy holds up in some ways. Physical activity can be mind-altering, affecting the same neurotransmitter systems as drugs like cannabis and cocaine. When exercisers claim to be junkies needing a fix, this high is surely part of what they're chasing. Exercise enthusiasts also display certain quirks more commonly associated with chemical dependence. Just as alcoholics are easily distracted by the presence of wine or liquor, people who exercise regularly show an attentional bias toward anything related to working out. This phenomenon—known as *attention capture*—reveals a brain always looking for an opportunity to indulge a favored habit. Even more compelling parallels can be seen in neuroimaging studies. For example, when self-proclaimed exercise addicts view images of people working out, their brains' craving circuitry fires up in a manner identical to what happens when you show cigarettes to a smoker. A small percentage of exercisers also show symptoms of psychological dependence, agreeing with statements such as "Exercise is the most important thing in my life" and "Conflicts have arisen between me and my family and/or my partner about the amount of exercise I do." One forty-six-year-old long-distance runner told researchers that she ran on a broken ankle for two years rather than take the rest needed to let the bones heal. Asked if anything could keep her from running, she said, "I suppose I could stop if somebody put shackles on me."

These studies suggest that physical activity taps into the same capacity to get hooked as the most powerfully habit-forming substances. Considering the similarities between exercise and addiction can help us understand how physical activity changes the brain. It also helps explain why physical activity becomes more rewarding the more you do it. However, there are limits to the exercise-addiction analogy. Most exercise enthusiasts are not suffering from a dependence that interferes with their health or the rest of their lives. What they have, instead, is a relationship with exercise that involves desire, need, and commitment. When it comes to the passion people profess for their favorite physical activity, there may be better comparisons than substance abuse. The fact that people get hooked on exercise is not, in the end, a classic story of addiction. If exercise is a drug, the one it most closely resembles is an antidepressant. And for many of us—myself included—getting hooked on exercise points not to its inherently addictive nature, but to our brain's capacity to latch onto a relationship that is good for us.

• • •

For more than a decade, scientists have been trying to develop a pill that mimics the physiological benefits of exercise. Instead of working out, you would ingest a drug that produces many of the same molecular changes in your body as strenuous training. Not everyone is convinced this is a worthwhile pursuit; biologist Theodore Garland Jr. told a *New Yorker* journalist, "Personally, I've been more interested in the possibility of drugs that would make us more motivated to exercise." Garland isn't the only scientist to raise this idea. Exercise physiologist Samuele Marcora has proposed the use of psychoactive drugs to encourage people to be more active. The most promising candidates, he argues, would be caffeine, followed by modafinil, a tablet that keeps people with narcolepsy awake, and methylphenidate, an amphetamine-like stimulant. Notably, these three drugs act primarily on dopamine and noradrenaline, two neurotransmitters who levels naturally rise during physical activity and contribute to its mood-boosting effects. Marcora has even suggested that drugs that target the opioid system could be useful if they enhanced an exercise high. ("I still remember the first horrified reaction of an exercise psychologist when I told him about this idea," Marcora writes.)

Whether this approach horrifies or intrigues you, it strikes me as overkill. It assumes that the human brain lacks the ability to find physical activity sufficiently rewarding and that it takes some other mind-altering substance to trick or tempt a person into liking exercise. But the research on this matter is clear: You don't need a psychoactive drug to make exercise habit-forming. In many ways, exercise *is* the drug. Like highly addictive substances, regular exposure to exercise will over time teach the brain to like, want, and need it.

All addictions start in the brain's reward system, and every drug of abuse—alcohol, cocaine, heroin, nicotine—acts on this system in a similar way. On first use, the drug triggers a flood of dopamine, the neurotransmitter that signals the presence of a reward. Dopamine grabs your attention and commands you to approach, consume, or do whatever set off the surge. Most drugs of abuse also increase other feel-good brain chemicals, like endorphins, serotonin, or noradrenaline. This powerful neurochemical combination is what makes a substance addicting.

Chronic use of such a drug eventually flips what researchers call the molecular switch for addiction. After repeated exposure to any habit-forming drug, a protein that helps the brain learn from experience accumulates inside neurons in the reward system. These proteins trigger long-lasting changes in dopaminergic brain cells that make them even more responsive to the substance that originally set off this process. In a regular cocaine user, the opportunity to use cocaine (and only cocaine) will trigger a tsunami of dopamine. For a heroin user, the possibility of taking heroin will set off a similar surge. In this way, consuming a drug teaches your brain to want it more.

Brains cells that have been sensitized in this way also become less responsive to other rewards; they have chosen their master. Try to tempt them with anything else and they will hold out. A cocaine-exposed reward system wants cocaine, not a home-cooked meal or a beautiful sunset. Once this molecular switch flips, all the signs of addiction set in. You will desire that reward over all others, become willing to sacrifice to obtain it, and suffer withdrawal if you cannot get it. This is the neurological path by which a short-lived pleasure ("This feels good!") becomes a stable desire ("I want this!") and eventually dependence ("I need this!").

Scientists have observed these changes in brains that have learned, through regular indulgence, to crave cocaine, alcohol, and sugar. But what about exercise? The answer is complicated. In some—but not all—ways, physical activity clearly resembles a habit-forming drug. Exercise causes the brain to release many of the same neurochemicals as addictive substances, including dopamine, noradrenaline, endocannabinoids, and endorphins. With repeat exposure, running also flips the molecular switch of addiction. In laboratory studies with rats, running ten kilometers a day for one month had an effect on dopaminergic neurons similar to that of a daily dose of cocaine or morphine. Wheel-running rats also demonstrate behaviors similar to those of addicted humans; if they are blocked from their wheels for twenty-four hours, they go on running binges when access is restored.

There are, however, important differences between exercise and drugs like cocaine. One has to do with timing. Although you see similar changes in the brain's reward system after exposure to exercise and drugs like cocaine, it takes longer to get hooked on exercise. Two weeks of wheel-running is insufficient to flip the molecular switch in laboratory rats, but after six weeks, rats run more each night and their brains show the neural signature of being hooked. Similarly, sedentary adults who begin high-intensity training show an increase in enjoyment over time, with pleasure peaking at six weeks. One study of new members at a gym found that the minimum "exposure" required to establish a new exercise habit was four sessions per week for six weeks. This delay in habit formation suggests that something different is happening, at a molecular level, than what occurs when a drug user becomes addicted. Drugs of abuse hijack the reward system and quickly take it over. Exercise seems instead to harness the reward system's ability to learn from experience in a more gradual way. As one woman who had avoided physical activity all her life, then surprised herself by becoming a runner and cyclist in her forties, told me, "Things change slowly. Sometimes you don't even recognize yourself as you're changing. Now I'm most happy when I'm in sneakers."

How you feel the first time you try a new form of exercise is not necessarily how you'll feel after you gain more experience.

For many, exercise is an acquired pleasure. The joys of an activity reveal themselves slowly as the body and brain adapt. One man, who his entire life had believed that he hated to exercise, told me that at age fifty-three, he decided to work with a personal trainer to improve his health and support his recovery in a twelve-step program. He started with one workout a week, and within three weeks, decided that he could tolerate a second weekly session. One day he left a training session and noticed that he was smiling, something he describes as shocking. "I realized that not only was I happy, I had found actual pleasure in my training session. I hadn't believed that kind of pleasure was possible outside of addiction."

For some people, it's a matter of finding the right activity at the right time—such as the young single mother who felt isolated and "like nothing more than a mum" until she joined a recreational netball league, found a network of friends, and discovered a new identity as an athlete. For others, it's about finding the movement their bodies were made for. One woman who started rowing in her forties told me, "So many of the women I row with thought they weren't athletes, but as soon as they got in the boat, their bodies said *yes*, and they found their home." Humans are also more psychologically complex than laboratory animals running in wheels. We get rewarded not just by how exercise feels, but also by what the activity means. One woman started going to the gym after leaving an abusive marriage. After thirty-eight years of having her movements constrained by her husband, she found being out in public and walking on a treadmill incredibly liberating. As she puts it, "I know I'm in freedom when I move."

Many people believe they don't enjoy exercise in any form, but I'd bet that most of them aren't immune to its rewards. It's possible that they just haven't exposed themselves to the dose, type, or community that would transform them into an "exercise person." When the right dose, type, place, and time come together, even lifelong abstainers can get hooked. Nora Haefele of Stowe, Pennsylvania, didn't start racing until her midfifties. Now sixty-two years old, she has completed more than two hundred events, including eighty-five half marathons. At her seventy-fifth half marathon, a race in Waterbury, Connecticut, the event director surprised her with a trophy, a golden sneaker with wings perched on a marble base with Haefele's name inscribed on it. That trophy now sits on a table in her living room, close to the rack that holds her finisher medals.

Haefele isn't fast. "Typically in a race, the gun goes off, and I'm alone within five minutes, and I'm alone until the end of the race," she says. She often crosses the finish line last, but she's found that most people cheer even harder for runners at the end of the pack. "I don't mind finishing last so someone else doesn't have to." She takes particular pride in persevering. At one half marathon in Harrisburg, it was raining so hard that the puddles were ankle deep and drivers were forced off the road. Haefele was the final runner to reach the finish line, but she earned first in her age group because everyone else in her category had backed out.

Haefele, a tax accountant, first started walking on a treadmill at work, but quickly realized that exercising indoors wasn't for her. She looked for something that would get her farther from her cubicle and discovered volkssporting, German for "the people's sports." Volkssporting takes a noncompetitive approach to outdoor walking, hiking, cycling, swimming, and cross-country skiing. You can show up at an event any time within the start-to-finish window, participate at your own pace, and take in the scenery and the company. Haefele started participating in 10K walks throughout the United States, enjoying both the travel and the people she met. To challenge her fitness more, she registered for her first timed race, a 5K walk. "When I signed up, I was terrified," she remembers. "I thought, *It's going to be all six-foot-tall twenty-year-olds, and they're going to look at me and say, 'What is that fat old woman doing here?'*" To her relief, it wasn't like that at all. She felt welcomed, finished the race, and realized, *I can do this.*

With more training under her belt, she signed up to walk a half marathon in Birmingham, Alabama, just "to see what it felt like." She was surprised to find that she enjoyed that, too, and decided to try running. "There have been times when I've been out there at mile ten, thinking, *Why did I think this is fun? This is horrible.* Other times I'm on cloud nine. I feel strong. I feel powerful. I'm accomplishing something. When I approach the finish line, I feel great." After Haefele passed the milestone of her seventy-fifth half marathon, she decided to aim for a hundred. "My races are a source of joy. At sixty-one, I feel privileged to feel that way."

When I asked Haefele if the races reminded her of anything, she instantly said, "Church. It's my way of celebrating the world. We're all out there celebrating, and sort of worshiping what's been given to us, and we're all grateful. It reminds me of a church service." After a pause, she added, "It's also like going to a rave. After a race, I'm in love with everybody, and sometimes it lasts the whole day. The person who's selling me a coffee at the convenience store on the way home, I'm like, 'I love that guy.' I've never done ecstasy, but that's how I imagine it is: All's well with the world, everybody's wonderful. If all you have to do is run thirteen miles to get that, it's so worth it." Haefele is a recovering alcoholic, and she hasn't had a drink since 1988. "This is now my drug of choice," she told me. "It fills the same need, but it does it in such a good way."

Haefele never expected to get hooked on racing. She was born in 1957 and went to school before Title IX, passed as part of the Education Amendments of 1972, which requires schools to offer the same athletic opportunities to girls and boys. "I always thought, 'Sports aren't for girls.' If you had told me in high school that at some point I'd be doing races, I would have thought you were insane. I thought I wasn't supposed to, that it wasn't for me. I was fat, too, and that makes you sometimes think, that world isn't for me, I'm not allowed to be there," she says. "Somewhere along the way, I thought, *Screw that. I'm going to go do stuff. Why am I limiting myself?* When you turn fifty, you stop worrying about other people. I don't know why I wasted my whole life thinking I wasn't allowed to do athletics because I was a girl and I was fat."

Now when Haefele hears that someone is thinking about trying a first 5K but is worried about finishing or belonging, she encourages them to take the risk. "I tell them the story about my first 5K, how afraid I was, and how it literally changed my life. If I can, I will offer to go with them," she says. "I like to throw in John Bingham's quote, 'The miracle isn't that I finished, it's that I had the courage to start.' I get weepy when I see that. If you can just find that little bit of courage that you need to start, it will change everything."

Whenever Nora Haefele drives past the exit for a race she has run, a warm and happy feeling floods her body. "I'll remember the day I did it, the weather, the people I saw, and how I felt when I finished," she told me. In 1976, marathon runner Ian Thompson told *New York* magazine, "I have only to think of putting on my running shoes and the kinesthetic pleasure of floating starts to come over me." Both Haefele's response to highway exits and Thompson's anticipatory runner's high point to one of the more curious similarities between addiction and exercise enthusiasm: the conditioned rush that scientists call the *pleasure gloss*. When you repeatedly experience a smell, sound, taste, sight, or touch in a context that is highly enjoyable, that sensation gets encoded in your memory of the pleasant experience. Eventually that sensation—even if it was originally neutral or unpleasant—becomes interpreted by the brain as highly pleasurable all by itself. Once this association is formed, ordinary sensory stimuli become pleasure bombs, setting off explosions of endorphins and dopamine. Consider, for example, the way NASCAR fans come to not just tolerate but savor the olfactory assault of burnt rubber. Or how a grown child whose parent baked still associates the whirring of a standing mixer with feeling safe and loved.

In the case of addiction, sensory cues can trigger powerful cravings or even withdrawal. The mere sight of drug paraphernalia or the smell of a place where someone has repeatedly gotten high can set off an intense desire to use. Psychiatrist Benjamin Kissin noted that when former heroin addicts returned to New York City after being incarcerated in Sing Sing for five years, they developed spontaneous withdrawal symptoms as soon as the train passed through their old neighborhoods.

Exercise enthusiasts report their own versions of the pleasure gloss and cue-dependent cravings. Sensations associated with exercise become highly pleasurable, and objects, places, or other cues related to a favorite activity can produce a strong desire to move. When I asked people I knew for their own examples, many offered odors: the chlorine of an indoor swimming pool, the scent of freshly cut grass on a soccer field, even the manure on a farm where one woman rides horses. A former student of mine said the smell of his yoga mat sets off his brain's pleasure circuit. When I asked what his mat smelled like, he said, "Rubbery chemicals," proof that the brain is willing to give anything a pleasure gloss. Other exercisers take satisfaction in sounds: the clank of heavy weights being dropped in the gym, the *pop!* of opening a can of tennis balls, or the click of cycling shoes locking into pedals. The source of pleasure could even be an object, such as the exercisers who recounted to me the gratification of a favorite running shirt ("When I put it on, I feel invigorated"), a yoga rug ("When I pack it into my bag the night before, I feel a sense of excitement for the next day . . . I definitely feel that happiness buzz when I touch the rug"), and a heart rate monitor ("When I plug it in to charge, I start to feel excited, in fact just thinking about it now is making my stomach have a few butterflies. When I have it in my hand, I feel a charge of empowerment"). How strange these statements must seem to the person who hasn't yet gotten hooked on any physical activity. I myself was surprised by how easily exercisers identified their own pleasure glosses. And yet these examples demonstrate just how genuine the reward of physical activity is. A brain makes such leaps and forms such associations only when the pleasure runs deep.

My own most deeply ingrained exercise-related anticipatory pleasure is the feel and sound of putting a VHS cassette in the VCR. I first discovered what was then called aerobics in the third grade when my mom started bringing home exercise videos she picked up at garage sales. At first she bought them for herself, imagining a future fitness kick that never materialized. I was the one who got hooked on the synthesized music and synchronized movements. In gym class and on the playground, I was uncoordinated, clumsy, and seemingly lacking in all athletic talent. But the workouts in these videos tapped into physical skills that no kickball game or shuttle run had ever called for: the ability to move to a musical beat and a knack for mirroring another person's movements. Doing these videos, I discovered the thrill of physical competence, so different from the humiliation of being unable to catch a ball or do a flip on the jungle gym bars. Doing leg lifts, I felt like a Rockette in the glamorous Radio City Music Hall Christmas Spectacular my grandparents had taken my sister and me to in New York City.

Much later on, when I became a psychologist, I would learn that the capacities to keep a beat and mirror other people's movements are both related to empathy. The workout videos tapped into the same personality trait that helped me lose myself in novels like *Julie of the Wolves* and kept me up at night worrying about the starving children we collected change for in UNICEF boxes. By doing so, calisthenics and dance aerobics gave me access to my body's intelligence in a way that competitive playground sports never had.

Over the years, I amassed quite a collection of tapes, stacking them up in the corner of the television room. (The original *Jazzercise* was a favorite of mine, in part because the instructor encouraged us to sing along as we danced and stretched.) I kept up a daily routine well into high school. Before each workout, I'd scan the stack, select a video, and slide it out of its cardboard case. After I inserted the video into the VCR, there'd be a satisfying click as the machine accepted the cassette, then the sound of the machine lifting the cassette's protective flap to expose the tape. By the time the TV screen came to life with the old FBI copyright infringement warning, my brain cells were awash in dopamine. I no longer have a VCR, but if you put one of my old aerobics videos in my hand, I'm sure my brain would remember the pleasure and my heart would beat faster in anticipation of step-touches to come.

Exercisers tend to experience these conditioned responses in a very different way than drug users who are trying to stay clean, perhaps because most feel no ambivalence about their habit. They welcome the cravings set off by a pleasure gloss and relish the way familiar sensations ignite their desire. These sensations are not triggers for an uncontrollable and self-destructive compulsion. Instead, for many exercisers, the pleasure gloss that coats ordinary sounds, smells, and objects serves to remind them of a long-standing and positive relationship they are grateful for. As one friend described his own pleasure gloss to me, "The martial arts academy where I've trained for fifteen years has a very unique smell—some combination of sweat, rubber from the mats, and Lord only knows what else. If I've been traveling for a bit and then return, my body reacts as if I've come home after being away a long time." His comment reminded me of the research showing that seeing a friend's face can set off the brain's reward system. That burst of dopamine and the subsequent rush of pleasure help solidify the relationship. Perhaps the same is true for each of the beloved sensations that exercisers savor. The feel of a favorite T-shirt's worn threads on your skin, the sound of a yoga mat unfurling and hitting hardwood floors, the mingling smells of sweat and wax as you step onto a basketball court—they deepen the pleasures inherent to movement and bond us more strongly to our activity of choice.

...

When my husband decided to train for a triathlon a couple of years ago, he started reading books and listening to podcasts about endurance sports. As he shared his favorite stories, one thing that stood out was how many of these athletes were in recovery from drug or alcohol addiction. Perhaps for some of them—such as the runner who compared the high of long-distance running to heroin—exercise is a substitute addiction. But it occurred to me that something else might be going on; that perhaps exercise can repair the neurological havoc wreaked by previous addictions.

Drugs of abuse would be far less destructive if all they did was teach your brain to want them. Their actual effects are more devastating, in part because when a substance unleashes an unnatural flood of feel-good chemicals, it triggers the brain's homeostatic mechanisms. Your brain will try to compensate for the drug's effects to keep your neurochemistry in balance. One way it does this is by activating the brain's anti-reward system, which works to dampen the effects of feel-good chemicals. The anti-reward system initially kicks in when the brain is flooded with abnormally high levels of dopamine or endorphins. The brain is attempting to reduce the extreme high, like pulling the plug in a bathtub so it doesn't overflow. When you regularly trigger the anti-reward system through repeated drug use, you teach the system to stay activated even when you aren't using. A brain that is used to being put in a state of extreme high will begin to kill your joy preemptively, producing a near-constant dysphoria. Chronic drug use also lowers the level of dopamine circulating in your brain and reduces the availability of dopamine receptors in the reward system. Both of these changes can leave you feeling unmotivated, depressed, antisocial, and unable to enjoy ordinary pleasures—a consequence neuroscientists have labeled the dark side of addiction.

Here's where the long-term effects of physical activity and substance abuse most dramatically diverge. Exercise produces a less extreme spike in dopamine, endorphins, and other feel-good chemicals. Drugs like cocaine or heroin wallop the system, but exercise merely stimulates it, leading to very different long-term adaptations. The brain reacts to regular exercise not by suppressing activity in the reward system, but by facilitating it. In direct contrast to drugs of abuse, exercise leads to higher circulating levels of dopamine and more available dopamine receptors. Instead of annihilating your capacity for pleasure, exercise expands it. The sensitization of the reward system to nondrug rewards such as food, social connection, beauty, and any number of ordinary pleasures may explain why exercise helps people recover from substance abuse. In both animal and human studies, physical activity reduces cravings for and abuse of cannabis, nicotine, alcohol, and morphine. In one randomized trial, adults in treatment for methamphetamine abuse participated in an hour of walking, jogging, and strength training three times a week. After eight weeks, their brains showed an increase in dopamine receptor availability in the reward system.

Studies like this suggest that exercise can reverse the anti-reward system's takeover of the brain and bring a numbed reward system back to life. In doing so, exercise resembles not so much a habit-forming drug of abuse as an antidepressant. The closest parallel I could find to how physical activity affects the reward system is not addiction, but continuous deep brain stimulation, one of the most promising medical treatments for depression. To prepare a patient for deep brain stimulation, a neurosurgeon drills a small hole into a patient's skull and slides an electrode into the patient's medial forebrain. The electrode is connected to a pulse generator surgically implanted in the patient's chest wall. The generator delivers continuous low-level voltage to the brain's reward system, much like a cardiac pacemaker regulates the beating of a patient's heart. Over time, deep brain stimulation remodels the reward system to make it more responsive and has been shown to cure even long-standing, treatment-resistant depression.

A meta-analysis of twenty-five randomized clinical trials concluded that exercise has a large and significant antidepressant effect among people diagnosed with major depressive disorder. Another review of thirteen studies—conducted in the U.S., the UK, Brazil, Germany, Norway, Denmark, Portugal, Italy, Spain, and Iran—found that adding exercise to treatment with antidepressant medication leads to larger improvements than medication only. While there are many ways physical activity can affect mood, its impact on the reward system almost certainly contributes to its antidepressant effects. One way to think about exercise is that it is a kind of do-it-yourself deep brain stimulation. When you exercise, you provide a low-dose jolt to the brain's reward centers.

Jump-starting the brain's reward system benefits not just those who suffer from depression or those who have struggled with drug abuse. Our brains change as we age, and adults lose up to 13 percent of the dopamine receptors in the reward system with each passing decade. This loss leads to less enjoyment of everyday pleasures, but physical activity can prevent the decline. Compared to their inactive peers, active older adults have reward systems that more closely resemble those of individuals who are decades younger. This may be one reason exercise is so strongly linked to happiness and a reduced risk of depression as we get older. It may also explain why people who eschewed exercise earlier in life find themselves drawn to it as they age. The same mind-altering properties that make the "drug" of movement an addictive pleasure to some makes it powerful medicine for others.

• • •

In 1993, Theodore Garland Jr.—the biologist who would, twenty-five years later, tell *The New Yorker* that he dreamed of a drug that could motivate people to exercise—started a selective breeding experiment with mice. Given access to wheels, mice will happily run, but Garland wanted to produce a genetic line that would run even more than the typical mouse. The earliest generations ran an average of four kilometers a day. By breeding only those mice who ran more than that, Garland's lab was able to select for and strengthen whatever genetic factors compelled them to run. By the fifteenth generation, Garland's mice were running fifteen kilometers a day. (A six-foot-tall man would have to run 168 miles a day to cover an equivalent distance for his body length.) Twenty-nine generations later, these selectively bred mice—known as "super-runners"—not only ran farther but also ran faster, ran more frequently, and took fewer breaks. If a lab assistant locked the running wheel so it would not rotate, the frustrated mice would climb the inside of the wheel in an attempt to run.

Garland's experiment had succeeded, but what biological

predispositions had his team exploited? One possible explanation is that the anatomy of the super-runners differed in a way that made running easier. It is true that as the breeding experiment progressed, super-runners began to show distinct physical traits, including more symmetrical thighbones and muscle cells that use energy more efficiently. But the early super-runners didn't have those attributes. Something else was motivating them to run. It turns out that the most notable distinction between normal mice and super-runners isn't in their muscles or their bones; it's in their brains. Specifically, the reward system. Super-runners have physically larger midbrains, including the structures of the reward system. They also show differences in gene expression and neurotransmitters throughout the reward circuit. This leads super-runners to get hooked on running more quickly than other mice. It takes less exposure to exercise to flip the brain's molecular switch of addiction, and they develop signs of cravings and dependence sooner. These mice are born to run not because they have the right bodies, but because they have the right brains. The original super-runners hadn't inherited an increased capacity to do the work of exercise; they had inherited an increased capacity to enjoy it. It was only through successive breeding that the super-runners' anatomy caught up with their brains, and they began to develop physical traits that supported their desire to run.

Reading about Garland's mice made me wonder: Are modern humans the equivalent of super-runners? Natural selection is a kind of selective breeding experiment. Some scientists argue that as the human species evolved, we developed a shared genome that reflects the survival advantage of being able, and willing, to exert ourselves. Maybe everything we know about how movement affects the human brain—from the runner's high to our ability to get hooked on exercise and the psychological benefits of being active—is proof that, whether or not we have a closet full of sneakers, humans are all, at some level, genetic super-runners.

And yet, there are also clear individual differences in how active people are. Could some humans exercise more because they have brains that are more easily hooked? There is evidence that the tendency to be active is at least partly heritable. By comparing identical twins raised together and apart, scientists have estimated that about 50 percent of the variability in physical activity is due to genetics. When you look at not just how much people exercise, but how much they enjoy it, heritability estimates drop to between 12 and 37 percent. That puts it on par with other psychological traits, like self-esteem (22 percent), empathy (27 percent), and fear of the dentist (30 percent), but much lower than physical traits like height and curliness of hair (both about 80 percent). Still, these numbers suggest a genetic influence. And, in fact, recent large-scale genome-wide association studies have identified dozens of genetic variants in humans that predict being more physically active. Some of these strands of DNA are on genes that influence metabolism, others are on genes linked to brain function, and still others remain a mystery—scientists aren't yet sure what roles they play in shaping human health or behavior.

I am utterly useless at team sports and was always one of the slowest runners in my class. But I fell hard for aerobics when I was eight, and I'm rarely as happy as I am when teaching group exercise. I was curious: Was this joy written in my genes? To find out, I ordered a DNA kit from 23andMe, drooled into a test tube, and shipped my saliva off to a processing center. The standard report didn't tell me anything about the strands of DNA that scientists have linked to exercise habits. However, when I clicked on "Raw Data," I discovered that I had access to every part of my genome that 23andMe had genotyped. As I entered each genetic identifier linked to physical activity into the search box, the results were mixed. I had many, but not all, of the variants associated with being more active. I wasn't sure how to interpret this. I had been hoping to discover a genetic profile that screamed, "Born to Move," but I realized I didn't actually know what this would look like. The genetic variants linked to being physically active are common, not rare. Movement was so key to our ancestors' survival that these mutations became broadly conserved across human populations.

Before I go further, I should acknowledge the profound limits of this investigation. Behavioral genetics is an emerging field, not settled science. Methods are constantly being improved and early findings discarded. Future work may uncover hundreds of genetic variants that shape how humans respond to exercise. Moreover, genes are not the whole story. There are many psychological, social, and environmental influences on human physical activity, far more than contribute to a rodent's wheel-running. I know this. And yet I felt compelled to interrogate my genes. I was sure that my love of exercise was, somehow, inborn and innate. That's because I have another source of data that has long convinced me that I was born to move: my identical twin sister, Jane, who not only shares my genes, but who also is just as committed to exercise as I am.

In early photographs, you cannot tell us apart unless one of us reveals the secret—I'm the one who usually looks like she's about to cry, while my sister looks like she is crafting some diabolical plan to take over the world. As adults, my sister and I are alike in many ways. We both touch our throats squeamishly at the mention of blood, and have a sweet tooth so strong we could thrive on a cane sugar IV drip. We both live in the San Francisco Bay Area despite growing up in suburban New Jersey, and we both married the men we started dating at age twenty-two. Our careers as researchers and writers have followed strikingly similar paths, and it's not uncommon for someone to tell me how much they love my work only to find out they are thinking of my sister. We are also both regular exercisers—it's as much a part of our lives as sleeping and eating. Jane is a distance runner who puts in between twenty-five and forty miles a week. She competes in an average of twelve races a year, including half and full marathons. When she gets near one of her favorite running trails, "I feel like a horse that's been in the stalls all week, antsy and stroking the ground with its front hooves, just raring to get out and gallop. I can't even ride in a cab past Central Park without wanting to leap out and do the six-mile loop."

I'll admit, I am mystified by her devotion to running, which has never appealed to me. She is equally confused by my love of group exercise. "I don't know how you get better," she told me, unsure why anyone would commit so much time to something you can't objectively improve at. "You don't have to get better," I countered. "You just enjoy it." But we are equally devoted to our preferred activities. While traveling, she scouts out running routes and races, and I look for the best place to take a group exercise class. On holidays and other special occasions, you'll find her with her husband and daughters at some themed 5K or half marathon, while I'll be teaching a community dance class. Moving is how we celebrate life. It is one of the most "twinny" things about us. Armed with this anecdotal evidence, I went back to the scientific literature, determined to figure out if there is anything else a human being can inherit that inclines them to get hooked on exercise. As it turns out, the answer is yes, and my sister and I have it: a genetic predisposition to experience the mental health benefits of physical activity.

Scientists have identified several strands of DNA, on multiple genes, that are linked to the antidepressant and anxiety-reducing effects of exercise. Individuals with any of these genetic variations seem to be more sensitive to the psychological benefits of regular exercise. For example, they are especially likely to show a reduced risk of depression and suicidal thinking if they exercise at least twenty minutes a day. As I searched for these genetic markers in my 23andMe data file, I discovered that my sister and I have all of them. My heart leapt at these results. No matter how fledgling the science might be, I couldn't help but be excited by what I was seeing. There is a possibility that our genes are peppered with nucleotides that make physical activity especially important for our mental well-being.

When I shared this discovery with my sister, she texted back, "Holy smokes! That's amazing!" And it is. Not just that exercise is good for mental health, but that our bodies and brains had independently guided us to something we both need. This has been especially true in recent years for my sister, who struggled with depression and suicidal thinking after a traumatic brain injury in our early thirties. Running has been one of the most effective and reliable ways she takes care of her mental health. "I am sure running does for me what antidepressants do for people for whom they work," my sister says. "If I've been sick or injured and haven't been able to run, as soon as I do my first run, I feel like the clouds have parted and the sun is shining, and I'm a human being again."

I feel the same way, except the darkness exercise protects me from is anxiety. I have always had a tendency toward worry. My parents generously called my early temperament *sensitive* and *shy,* but a more accurate description of me as a child would have been *scared.* I was the kid begging *not* to go on amusement park rides, who got sick to my stomach before math tests and birthday parties, and who nervously calculated how long our family's stockpile of Girl Scout cookies would last in a nuclear apocalypse (it was the early 1980s). I can dredge up no origin story, no childhood experience, that would explain this personality trait. All I've come up with is: I was born that way. I have a brain that expects calamity and is easily overwhelmed. If I had to guess my biologically determined psychological set point, I'd locate it somewhere between "on high alert" and "consumed by dread."

One theory of chronic worry is that people like me have an overactive fear circuit in our brains, set off not by anything specific, but operating more like constant background noise: *There's something wrong. There's something wrong.* The hyperactivity of this circuit produces a vague feeling of anxiety, leaving our imaginations to figure out what exactly we should be worried about. I can't say for sure that's what's happening in my brain, but it matches what I observe going on in my mind. And without a doubt, exercise has been the most powerful antidote I've discovered. Scientific research bears my experience out. A single dose of physical activity immediately decreases anxiety and rumination, and this effect becomes even more pronounced with regular exercise. A 2017 meta-analysis of exercise interventions found that physical activity can be an effective treatment for anxiety disorders.

When I was eight years old and first discovering the mood-altering effects of aerobics, none of today's commonly prescribed antianxiety or antidepressant drugs existed. It was rare for a child to be in therapy or to have access to any mental health guidance. In fact, I don't think it ever occurred to anyone that my mind was something that needed to be managed. Somehow I stumbled onto something that helped me handle the predispositions I was born with. There is something heartening about this revelation. I feel fortunate that my brain figured this out despite the fact that I lacked any natural athletic ability and grew up in a home where neither parent exercised nor played sports. I may not be a super-runner in the traditional sense, but this research helped me realize that there is more than one way to be born to move. My daily exercise habit doesn't so much sedate me as it emboldens me, which is exactly the right remedy for my anxiety. Being active makes me a better version of myself, and for this reason, I am grateful to be hooked.

The summer after I finished college, I joined a health club as a graduation gift to myself. My first week there, the club held a fair. Along with a prize wheel where you could win water bottles and guest passes, a chiropractor provided postural analyses and a psychic offered readings in a corner of the weight room. Curious as to what kind of advice I would get next to a bench press, I sat for a reading. The psychic took one look at me and told me to try the cardio kickboxing class. Maybe she could see the anxiety that coursed through my veins; maybe I was wearing it on my face. At the time I lived alone, in a studio apartment, and for the previous year, I had been carrying pepper spray in my purse and walking home from work with keys splayed between my fingers. I don't think the woman who guided me to kickboxing was psychic, but she gave me great advice. Those classes changed me. By the end of the summer, I learned how to land a hook, an uppercut, and a jab. I was used to clenching my hands into worried fists, but fists feel different when you're throwing punches. To this day, no other form of exercise makes me feel so powerful.

Here's something I've come to believe: Movement isn't addictive only when it feels pleasurable. I think the brain can sense resilience being wired in. And in fact courage is another predictable side effect of how physical activity changes the brain. At the very same time that a new exercise habit is enhancing the reward system, it also targets regions of the brain that regulate anxiety. In laboratory studies with rats, twenty-one days of running altered their brain stems and prefrontal cortexes—areas of the brain that control the body's response to fear and stress—in ways that made the rats braver and better able to handle stressful situations. In humans, exercising three times a week for six weeks increases neural connections among areas of the brain that calm anxiety. Regular physical activity also modifies the default state of the nervous system so that it becomes more balanced and less prone to fight, flight, or fright. The latest research even suggests that lactate, the metabolic by-product of exercise that is commonly, but erroneously, blamed for muscle soreness, has positive effects on mental health. After lactate is released by muscles, it travels through the bloodstream to the brain, where it alters your neurochemistry in a way that can reduce anxiety and protect against depression. I like to think that when I fell in love with kickboxing that summer twenty years ago, or even back when I slid my first aerobics tape into the VCR, my brain understood that a positive transformation was under way. Something deep in my DNA recognized a good thing, and said, *Yes, thank you, keep going.*

IN A LABORATORY EXPERIMENT at the University of Wisconsin, Madison, researchers set out to capture what happens in the brains of mice who love wheel-running but are denied the opportunity. Just before their nightly run, the researchers blocked each mouse's access to the running wheel. The mice were ready to exercise but couldn't—as if you had shown up at the gym excited to work out, only to find the doors locked and the lights off. In that moment of thwarted desire, each mouse was sacrificed. The researchers scooped out its brain, slicing and staining the gray matter for examination. Under a microscope, they observed chemical evidence that the mouse had been in a state of heightened longing when it died. Areas of the brain associated with desire, motivation, frustration, and even the physical initiation of running were coactivated. This pattern is similar to what you'd see in a smoker craving a cigarette but not allowed to smoke. But you could just as easily liken it to a homesick child missing his mom or a widow staring at the now-empty side of the bed.

The word *addict* comes from the Latin *addictus*, meaning both "devoted" and "bound to." Some neuroscientists have mused that all devotions—between lovers or between caregiver and child—are a kind of addiction. They point to similarities in the brain between adoration and dependence. When heartbroken young adults see a photo of their beloved, their brains instantly shift into a state resembling an addict's cravings for cocaine. When a mother gazes at her baby, her brain's reward system becomes activated in a way that neuroscientists compare to a drug high. The scent of her infant's skin can trigger a neural response close to hunger. (One of my favorite headlines describing this research comes from the *Daily Mail Australia*, which assured readers, "Your compulsion as a mum to eat your baby is totally normal.")

However, the tendency to view love through the language of

substance abuse can lead to unsatisfying analogies. One research paper described missing a loved one as "withdrawal" and the desire to reunite a "relapse." These analyses make it seem like the primary function of the reward system is to addict, and anything that taps into this system is merely exploiting that capacity. But why assume that addiction is the phenomenon that all other devotions mimic? From an evolutionary standpoint, this makes no sense. Cocaine isn't why the reward system exists; the drug just happens to stimulate it exceptionally well. Moreover, the reward system is, evolutionarily speaking, ancient. In all manner of creatures, dopamine motivates behaviors that are key to survival: eating, mating, and caregiving. The reward system's main job is not to make us dependent on things that are harmful, but to push us toward the things we actually need.

In humans, that includes other people. And when you fall in love or become a caregiver, the reward system helps you forge strong attachments so that you will stay together. Through the repeated pleasure you experience from contact with loved ones, you come to like, crave, and need these relationships. You become willing to sacrifice to maintain them. When you are separated, you long to be reunited. This isn't a destructive dependence; it's a neurobiological mechanism for commitment. The same brain responses that scientists compare to addiction are also signs of strong bonds. The burst of dopamine in a mother's brain when she sees her infant predicts her ability to bond with and soothe her child. In long-term happily married couples, a dopamine surge upon seeing your spouse is linked to how much you view their well-being as integral to your own. And when a widow or widower in the throes of grief sees a photo of their spouse, the activity of the reward system correlates with their self-reported yearning for their loved one.

Maybe it is more accurate to think of *commitment*, not addiction, as the primary function of the reward system. Perhaps it is this capacity that exercise taps into. From this view, our ability to get hooked reflects our tendency to get attached. Physical activity isn't just another habit-forming drug; instead, it harnesses our capacity to form the kind of bonds that hold together our most important relationships. As we've seen, exercise doesn't impair your reward system the way destructive addictions do. What's becoming clearer is that physical activity changes your brain in ways that are similar to having a child or falling in love. For example, new mothers and fathers show an increase in gray matter in the reward system during their first few months of caregiving. The more this part of the brain expands, the more the parents describe their babies as beautiful and perfect and themselves as blessed. This neurological change—a boost to the reward system—looks a lot like what happens when people develop an exercise habit. And the ultimate result is not so different from what humans experience when they form close attachments. By harnessing the brain's capacity to fall in love, regular exercise helps us joyfully commit to a relationship that enriches our lives and augments our happiness.

Chapter 3

COLLECTIVE JOY

At the oldest rowing club in Canada, the masters women's crew meets after work to train. Their teamwork starts on land, as the women carry an eight-seat racing shell on their shoulders to the Ottawa River on the edge of the Canadian Shield. As they move from the boathouse to the water, the odors of rotting wood, epoxy, and old sports equipment are replaced by fresh air and the fragrance of forest trees.

The rowers face backward in the water, and as they head upstream, they can't see where they are going. They depend on the coxswain, who sits at the stern, to steer and call directions. The women also rely on their ability to sense the winds, the boat, the water, and one another. No one except the coxswain speaks. Every rower has her own blade, which they move in and out of the water in unison. With each synchronized stroke, the boat is lifted up by all eight blades and vaulted over the surface of the river. In that moment of gliding, there's a swooshing sound of water rushing under the boat—a sound so satisfying, the women on the crew call it "rowing cocaine." To accomplish this move, the rowers must be completely in sync. Any subtle resistance to the rhythm and swing of the stroke interrupts the flow of the racing shell over the water.

"It's total attunement," says Kimberly Sogge, one of the women on the crew of over-fifty athletes. "We're all feeling each other and the movement of the water, and it becomes not clear who is feeling what, because we're one living entity. Not just with one another, but also the river." Sometimes the crew stops on the water in the middle of a training session to look around, breathe, and listen. Sogge savors these moments. "When the light is in such a way that the boundaries between the water and sky have dissolved, and we have been in this rhythm where the boundaries between us as humans have dissolved—that is ultimate bliss. I can't imagine heaven is some other place."

The feeling Sogge describes is not reserved for rowing. It can be experienced anytime and anywhere people gather to move in unison: in marches or parades, at dance classes and night-clubs, while jumping rope on the sidewalk or practicing tai chi in the park, or when swaying and singing at church. In 1912, French sociologist Émile Durkheim coined the term *collective effervescence* to describe the euphoric self-transcendence individuals feel when they move together in ritual, prayer, or work. Durkheim believed that these activities help individuals feel connected to one another and to something bigger than themselves. We crave this feeling of connection, and synchronized movement is one of the most powerful ways to experience it.

The joy of collective effervescence helps explain why fitness friendships and sports teams feel like family; why social movements that include physical movement inspire greater solidarity and hope; and why individuals feel empowered when they join others to walk, run, or ride for a cure. As with the runner's high, our capacity for collective effervescence is rooted in our need to cooperate to survive. The neurochemistry that makes moving in unison euphoric also bonds strangers and builds trust. This is why moving together is one of the ways humans come together. Collective action reminds us what we are part of, and moving in community reminds us where we belong.

•••

The Brazilian island of Marajó lies at the mouth of the Amazon River. On that island, in a village called Soure, psychology graduate student Bronwyn Tarr lay awake in a bed-and-breakfast, sweating under a mosquito net in the dark. She was exhausted but too jet-lagged to sleep. Through the thin walls, she heard her research assistant next door zapping mosquitoes. Tarr could also make out the sound of drumbeats somewhere in the distance. Intrigued, she got out of bed, tied a sarong around her waist, and grabbed a flashlight. She followed the sound along dusty roads pocked with potholes. She could smell meat cooking and the scent of mangoes hanging from trees, but no one else seemed to be out. The only creatures she encountered were wandering buffaloes attracted to the ripe fruit.

After walking a while, she came to a building with the lights on. The windows and doors were flung open and music spilled out. Tarr, who didn't know how to say anything other than *olá* in Portuguese, hesitated near the door. A young man spotted her, smiled, and gestured for her to come in. The room was packed with teenagers and adults dancing the carimbó, a folkloric dance of the island. Live musicians played the drums, flute, and guitar, and women danced in pairs, holding their skirts and turning in circles. One woman, seeing Tarr on the sidelines, grabbed her by the wrist and pulled her in. Tarr did her best to follow along, mimicking the woman's moves. At the end of the song, her partner bowed to thank her. It didn't matter that Tarr was an outsider or that she didn't speak the language. She felt like she belonged, and she stayed to dance for hours.

Tarr could hardly have scripted a more fitting welcome to the village. She and her research assistant had traveled to Marajó Island to study how dance brings people together. She was particularly interested in the sense of unity and self-transcendence people often report when dancing in groups. When I asked Tarr how she would describe the feeling to someone who had never experienced it, she struggled for words. Instead, she made a gesture, turning her palms to the sky and looking up. "It centers from here," she said, touching her chest over her heart. "It feels expansive, even though it's internal. The boundary of who you are dissolves."

This feeling—what modern researchers refer to as *collective joy*—is the main reason I love group exercise. I experience it both when I teach and when I take class as a student. But Tarr is right; it's a tricky thing to explain. The best description I've found comes not from a psychologist or a dancer, but from British anthropologist A. R. Radcliffe-Brown, who spent time in the early twentieth century observing the indigenous people of the Andaman Islands in the Bay of Bengal, east of India. The islanders engaged in frequent dance rituals, and Radcliffe-Brown was particularly impressed by the rituals' psychological effects:

> As the dancer loses himself in the dance, as he becomes absorbed in the unified community, he reaches a state of elation in which he finds himself filled with energy or force immensely beyond his ordinary state, and so finds himself able to perform

prodigies of exertion. This state of intoxication, as it might almost be called, is accompanied by a pleasant stimulation of the self-regarding sentiment, so that the dancer comes to feel a great increase in his personal force and value. And at the same time, finding himself in complete and ecstatic harmony with all the fellow-members of his community, experiences a great increase in his feelings of amity and attachment towards them.

Radcliffe-Brown also noted one aspect of the ritual that psychologists like Bronwyn Tarr suspect is the key to producing collective joy: *synchrony*. The Andamans all performed the same simple dance step at the same time to one beat, generated by a man stomping his foot on a wooden sounding board. Even when a dancer needed to rest, he would continue to lift and lower one heel at a time to keep the beat.

While on Marajó Island, Tarr ran an experiment with local high school students to help tease apart the psychological effects of music, dancing with others, and moving in synchrony. The students danced in groups to music. Some of the groups were given steps to perform in unison, while others did not coordinate their moves. Afterward, the students who had danced in unison felt more bonded to their fellow group members than the students who had danced together, but not in synchrony. When Tarr returned to the UK, she repeated this experiment in a series of silent discos, where participants danced to music delivered through headphones. Once again, those who moved in unison felt more strongly connected to the strangers they had danced with. Music and physical exertion can play a role in collective joy, but synchrony is the most crucial component.

Tarr knew that endorphins, the brain's natural pain relievers, can produce both euphoria and social bonds among strangers, so she also measured dancers' ability to tolerate pain. (She did this by strapping a blood pressure cuff on each participant's upper arm and inflating it until they could no longer stand the discomfort. I was skeptical that this method could generate significant pain, so I ordered a blood pressure cuff online and tried it. I am no longer skeptical.) Once again, it was the dancers who moved in synchrony who showed the strongest increase in pain tolerance. When Tarr gave dancers a 100-milligram dose of naltrexone, a drug that blocks the effects of endorphins, synchronized movement did not increase their ability to withstand pain. This finding confirmed that collective joy is driven in part by endorphins.

We usually associate an endorphin rush with high-intensity exercise, but Tarr has found that calm synchronized movement, even small gestures done while sitting, will also increase pain tolerance and social closeness among strangers. One place you can experience this is in a flow yoga class, when practitioners synchronize both their movements and their breathing. The breath becomes the beat that drives the flow of poses, and the sound of the group inhaling and exhaling in unison provides a satisfying sensory feedback. Studies show that yoga, like dancing, can create social bonds. In one experiment, strangers who practiced yoga together reported a sense of connection and trust with the other members of the group. Afterward, when that group played an economic game, they cooperated more than groups who had engaged in a less synchronized activity.

I taught group yoga classes for years, and I remember well the sense of togetherness it can produce. Walking to my regularly scheduled yoga class on September 12, 2001, I wondered if anyone would show up, or if everyone had been so traumatized and disoriented by the previous day's events that the room would be empty. But students arrived on time and unrolled their mats. Many were quieter than usual. One woman lay down in relaxation pose and didn't get up until the end of class. I led the group through a familiar flow, the sequence we had practiced every week for months. I used as few words as possible and relied on our collective muscle memory to carry us through. We moved and breathed together, first through sun salutations, then standing poses. As we held each posture, I heard myself say over and over, "Inhale. Exhale." The synchronized poses and breathing worked their magic, but the flood of endorphins that day served a different role. Not euphoric bliss, but relief. For ninety minutes, we didn't fall apart, and for ninety minutes, no one was alone. It was another kind of collective joy. A salve. Whatever fear, confusion, or sadness we felt as individuals was held by something bigger, and in that space, we found room to breathe.

When psychologist Bronwyn Tarr tried to describe the feeling of collective joy, she emphasized the sense of self and other merging: "The boundary of who you are dissolves." Kimberly Sogge used the same language to describe the bliss of rowing with her crew on the Ottawa River: "We have been in this rhythm where the boundaries between us as humans have dissolved." The feeling of boundaries dissolving is one of the most powerful aspects of collective joy. It's not the *idea* of being connected; it is a physical *sensation* of connection. Somehow the brain is tricked into perceiving your body as just one part of a larger whole that it can sense in its entirety.

To explain how moving in synchrony produces this effect, Tarr likes to demonstrate a psychological trick called the *rubber hand illusion*. Imagine sitting at a table and resting both of your arms on the tabletop. An experimenter conceals your right arm and replaces it with a rubber arm. When you look down, you see your own left arm and the fake rubber arm where your right arm should be. The experimenter then strokes the rubber arm with a paintbrush, which you can see, while simultaneously stroking your real right arm out of view, which you can feel. Your brain simultaneously receives these two sensations: the feeling of your real arm being touched by the paintbrush and the sight of the paintbrush stroking the rubber arm. When these two streams reach your sensory cortex at the same time, the synchrony of their arrival produces the illusion that the rubber arm is part of you. Even though, intellectually, you know it is fake, you will look at the rubber arm and think, *That is a part of me*. You won't just *think* it. You will *sense* it. The illusion is so strong that if the experimenter was to pick up a pair of scissors and stab the rubber arm, you would scream and push back from the table.

This is how synchronized movement works, too, to create the sensation of group unity. As you move, your brain receives feedback from your muscles, joints, and inner ear about what your body is doing. Simultaneously, you see others performing the same movements. When these inputs arrive at once, your brain merges them into one unified perception. The movements you see in others become linked to the movements you feel, and your brain interprets the other bodies as an extension of your own. The more fully the brain integrates these perceptual streams, the more connected you feel to those you are moving with. Neuroscientist and dancer Asaf Bachrach calls this the *kinaesthetics of togetherness*. This phenomenon may even extend to the objects we move with; one kayaker described to me feeling that her kayak was an extra limb of her body. A sailor who reported a similar sensation with his sailboat concluded that is why people love their boats so much.

The perception of a collective self also alters your sense of personal space, the area around you that feels like it belongs to you. When a person's sense of self transfers to some other object (like a rubber hand) or to a bigger group, that individual's sense of personal space transfers, too. When Bronwyn Tarr says that the essence of collective joy is an expanded sense of self, this is part of what she's describing. Your understanding of the part of the world that belongs to you expands, too. This feeling can translate into both self-confidence and social ease. You can walk away from a dance party or group exercise class with an expanded sense of belonging and an embodied knowing that you have the right to take up space in the world.

More than once it has occurred to me how fortunate I am to have become a group exercise instructor when I was only twenty-two years old. Teaching group exercise was the first environment I ever felt so at ease and accepted in. Every day I taught class, I could walk into a room and be greeted by individuals who were genuinely happy to see me. The participants in these classes seemed to like me so much more, in such a reflexive way, than anything I'd ever experienced. They smiled when I ran into them on campus or around town. They gave me rides to the airport and offered to help me move to a new apartment. They told me stories about their lives and let me share in celebrating their milestones. Teaching group exercise, I felt welcomed, over and over and over again. I can't even begin to explain how extraordinary a gift that was. The sense of belonging carried over into every aspect of my life, undermining my social anxieties and my tendency to isolate myself in times of stress.

It would be years before I'd learn the neuroscience that explains why my students saw the best in me. When you lead people in movement, a group-level trust is cultivated, but you, the instructor, are the one constant beneficiary of any synchrony-based bonding. Every person in the room has the experience of watching and synchronizing with you. The hours my students spent mimicking my movements contributed to a felt sense, in their bodies, that they could trust me. This trust was, in a way, unearned. I had unintentionally exploited a social shortcut. But the trust of my students had a very real impact on me. Scientists who study social relationships have discovered that trust is a self-fulfilling prophecy. People who are viewed as trustworthy act in more generous and dependable ways. This becomes further evidence of their trustworthiness, and people trust them even more.

At a very formative time in my life, I stumbled into this upward spiral of social trust, based purely on the fact that I led groups moving in unison. I am sure that this shaped who I am today. When someone views you through a positive lens, you tend to rise to those expectations. It's as if you are being given permission to be your best self. Over the years, I was able to grow into the version of myself that my students perceived: someone who genuinely cares about them and our community, and someone who will happily contribute to the collective good. These traits were already inside me. They are part of what drew me to group exercise. Yet would they have had the same space to develop if I hadn't stepped into the instructor's role? Would I have become someone who sees the good in others if I hadn't first benefited from my students' positive projections? It's a remarkable privilege, to be on the receiving end of so much collective joy. I wish that every person could experience it.

• • •

In March 2016, CrossFit gym owner Brandon Bergeron received notice that the property housing his gym in Grass Valley, California, had been sold. He needed to vacate the premises immediately. Devastated, Bergeron let his members—who had become a community by lifting, squatting, and sweating together—know. They responded to the news by showing up with three pickup trucks and a U-Haul to help Bergeron move out. As he told a reporter for the local paper *The Union*, "A whole gym that took three years to build, every nut and bolt was gone in eight hours." When he found a new location two months later, the community turned out again to help rebuild the gym.

One of the side effects of collective joy—along with the elation, ecstatic harmony, and affection heralded by anthropologist A. R. Radcliffe-Brown—is cooperation. Because synchronized movement increases trust, it encourages us to share and help out. Studies show that after walking in step with someone, tapping to the same beat, or even just moving a plastic cup side to side in unison, people cooperate more in an economic game, sacrifice more to benefit the greater good, and are more likely to help a stranger. Even babies show this effect. When fourteen-month-olds are bounced to music, facing an experimenter who bounces in sync, they are more likely to later help that experimenter pick up dropped markers. In some basic and primal way, when we move together, we tie our fates together, and we become invested in the well-being of those we move with.

Anthropologists believe that this may be the most important function of collective joy: to strengthen the social ties that encourage cooperation. Some liken it to the social grooming of chimpanzees, baboons, and gorillas, who pick ticks and fleas off one another, brush away dirt, and work out tangles in fur. Such grooming is not primarily about hygiene or appearance. It's a way to bond. The social touch leads to an endorphin rush that strengthens the animals' relationship and leads to real alliances. Primates who groom one another are more likely to share food and defend one another during a conflict.

Endorphins are especially effective at strengthening ties to individuals we are not related to. This is true not just in other primates, but also among people. Repeated exposure to endorphins while in the company of others builds an extended family. We humans have our own forms of social grooming, including shared laughter, singing, dancing, and storytelling. (Anthropologists think this is the likely order that these social behaviors first appeared in human history.) All of these activities release endorphins, and because you can laugh, sing, dance, and tell stories with many people at once, these group forms of social grooming make it possible to build large social networks with less time invested. And that's a good thing, because humans thrive when our social networks are broad and diverse.

Across cultures, most people's social networks can be described by five widening circles of connection. The first, innermost circle typically has only one other person in it, a primary life partner. The second circle contains close family and friends, with an average of five members. These are the people who would be devastated if something happened to you and would make significant sacrifices to help you. The next circle is the core friendship circle. It includes, on average, fifteen people who play an important role in your life. You would invite these friends or family members to special gatherings, and you could comfortably call on them for favors. The next circle includes fifty or so individuals that you could describe as friends, but have less close ties to. The outermost circle contains about one hundred and fifty people you are connected to in more casual ways at work, in your local community, through organizations you belong to, or by the activities you participate in.

It is the outer two circles that are most likely to get populated and strengthened through the social grooming of collective joy, whether through synchronized movement, singing, or shared laughter. And these outer circles, when robust, provide the kind of social support that can keep us going in small but meaningful ways. Kimberly Sogge of the Ottawa Rowing Club told me that the way rowers attune with one another on the boat translates into a quiet but effective community of mutual care. "When someone's in trouble, just like when you're rowing, you don't announce it, but somehow the message gets communicated and people start doing things. The farmer will bring honey or kale. People really notice each other and what you need appears."

Émile Durkheim believed the collective effervescence experienced in religious activities was one of the core social functions of church. It helped to create communities committed to group life. Modern religious scholars note that fitness communities have come to serve a similar role for many. Casper ter Kuile and Angie Thurston, fellows at Harvard Divinity School, observed CrossFit communities across the United States. They concluded that the local gyms, called "boxes," were functioning like community hubs, similar to places of worship, where people looked out for one another. CrossFit regulars drove fellow members to medical appointments, delivered meals to members whose spouse or close relative was sick, and even raised money, or helped find work, for members in need.

I heard one such account from Caroline Kohles, the senior director of fitness and wellness at the Marlene Meyerson Jewish Community Center in Manhattan. Kohles teaches Nia, a movement form that integrates dance, martial arts, and yoga. One of Kohles's regular Nia students, Susan, had recently lost her husband, Henry, after fifty years of marriage. Susan decided to honor Henry's wishes by not having any formal burial, ceremony, or memorial. Kohles told me, "He was cremated, and without that ritual, she was left sitting home alone. I went to visit Susan and told her, 'When you come back to class, we will do a special class in his honor.'" Henry loved classical music, so Kohles started putting together a playlist of pieces they could dance to: Claude Debussy's "Clair de Lune," the molto allegro from Mozart's Symphony no. 14, Vivaldi's Concerto in E Major, "Spring."

The day Susan returned, about two weeks after Henry passed, it happened to be a student's birthday. Another woman in class was celebrating her son's marriage. These are all things Kohles would usually acknowledge. She remembers thinking, *How do you honor a wedding, a funeral, and a birthday in one class?* She chose to play "Lean on Me" by Bill Withers as the last song, and asked the group to form a circle. Kohles first invited the birthday woman to come into the center to be celebrated. Then she called in the woman whose son was getting married, so the group could share her joy. Finally the entire class held hands in the circle and placed the memory of Henry in the middle. "We swayed, pulsed, held hands, lifted our hearts and hands up, and sent Henry off on his final journey." Afterward, a group of students honored Susan and Henry with an impromptu shivah. They purchased coffee, fruit, and breakfast rolls, and listened as Susan told stories about her life with Henry. "We'll take care of Susan," Kohles said. "We'll make sure she comes to the gym and support her as she reenvisions her life." When I checked in with Kohles more than a year later, she shared that Susan still comes to class regularly. Every once in a while, Kohles plays Henry's classical music playlist, always in honor of Susan and Henry.

For much of human history, the size and membership of your social network was limited by geography. Now family can be halfway around the world, and through technology, we can connect with strangers anywhere on the planet. As our social circles widen and disperse, it's worth asking: Is it possible to experience collective joy at a distance—moving at the same time, if not in the same place—to create a community that is not bounded by proximity?

The Exertion Games Lab, a research group at RMIT University in Melbourne, Australia, designed the Jogging over a Distance app to connect two runners in different locations. The users talk by phone as they jog, and the app uses each runner's GPS to determine their pace. When you keep pace with your partner, their voice sounds like they are right next to you. If you run faster, the app makes their voice sound like it's coming from behind you. In this way, the app encourages runners to synch up. (You can also use heart rate to calculate pace, so that "in sync" is determined by effort, not objective speed.) The spatialized audio feedback creates a more realistic sense of running side by side than simply chatting over the phone. As one early user of the technology said, "I felt like he was there with me."

Other technologies connect users to a much bigger community. Jennifer Weiss, a forty-eight-year-old orthopedic surgeon in Southern California, rides her Peloton stationary bike in her garage at five-thirty most mornings. The bike connects her to as many as eight hundred riders around the world through a video app, which streams a live workout from Peloton's New York City studio. The app also sends data about Weiss's performance to the instructor and a community leaderboard, where every rider is listed according to their bike's speed and resistance. When Weiss is near someone on the leaderboard and sees their place rise and fall in relationship to hers, it feels like she is physically riding with them in a pack. When the instructor tells participants to ride to the beat of the music, Weiss knows that riders all over the world are cycling at the exact same cadence. This part of the ride reminds her of the feeling she gets in a flow yoga class when everyone is moving and breathing in unison.

In both of these cases—Jogging over a Distance and the livestreamed Peloton classes—technology enables genuine connection. But technology can also be used to simulate social interaction. The same Exertion Games Lab that built the Jogging over a Distance app also created Joggobot, the world's first robotic jogging companion. Joggobot is essentially a surveillance drone. You tell the robot in advance what path you plan to run, and it uses GPS to follow that route. You wear a T-shirt with a target on your chest so that the quadcopter's camera can detect you. Joggobot watches you run and flies ten feet ahead to keep you company. In early tests of the device, joggers quickly embraced the robot as a running mate. They easily and instinctively humanized the quadcopter, interpreting its whirring noise as a sign of exertion, as if Joggobot were breathing hard and struggling to keep up. When sensor errors or wind made

Joggobot veer off course, the joggers interpreted it as "having a mind of its own."

How to think about this? If your primary goal is to harness the human desire for companionship to make exercise more enjoyable, Joggobot is genius. But what if authentic social connection is the true need, and being active is a way to fulfill it? You could argue that anyone who craves connection would reject Joggobot and join a running group or head to the local YMCA. But it can be intimidating to show up in a new space. Rather than take that risk, maybe you would decide to go for a walk with your drone or settle for a virtual reality glove that rapidly compresses to makes it feel like you were just high-fived by a workout partner.

Bronwyn Tarr has recently replicated her dance experiments in virtual reality, and when people dance with an avatar, they like the avatars who dance in sync with them more than the avatars who do their own thing. They also experience the same increases in pain tolerance as people dancing with other humans in a shared physical space. These results suggest that virtual reality can give you the same endorphin rush as authentic social synchrony. I admit that this finding surprised me. Then again, it's probably part of why, growing up, I had such a positive response to exercise videos. It also helps explain why dance video games that require you to synchronize with an avatar are so popular. They tap into a very real neurochemical reward. Virtual reality will make the illusion of synchronized connection even more convincing—and yet I'm left feeling ambivalent about that progress. If collective joy evolved as a form of social grooming, those endorphins aren't released just to make you feel good. They're supposed to nurture important relationships and help you develop a social support network.

When you move with an avatar or a robot, what relationship does that endorphin rush benefit?

Technology that exploits our social instincts won't necessarily provide the same benefits as the experience it mimics. When my sister's twin daughters were born two months premature, she and her husband moved into the neonatal intensive care unit. Among the many events they missed, they couldn't make a 10K trail race they had registered for. Their running group picked up their race bibs and talked the organizers into handing over the medals my sister and her husband would have received if they had finished the race. The running group sent them the bibs and medals and said, "Go run a 10K wherever you are." As my sister recalls, "We pinned on our bibs, ran a 10K around the hospital, wore the medals the rest of the day, and sent photos to the group. It was a time in our lives when everything was out of control and so overwhelming. We felt very embraced by the runners who did that for us." Do I even need to pose the rhetorical question of whether Joggobot would be there for them in the same way?

I don't pretend to know where the line lies between authentic connection and simulation. These are questions the fields of artificial intelligence and virtual reality are grappling with, as sex robots and caregiver robots and pet robots become feasible alternatives to their carbon-based counterparts. Soon we'll all have to decide where our own line is, and in domains far more intimate than jogging buddies. As we are pushed in every aspect of our lives toward technological connectivity as opposed to shared space and direct contact, activities that put us in the physical presence of others may become increasingly rare and especially important. Even people who enjoy bonding over technology need close-to-home connection. I couldn't help but smile when

Peloton enthusiast Jennifer Weiss told me that she bought a second bike so that her husband can ride alongside her. Some of her favorite rides are when their three young kids join the two of them in the garage and dance to keep them company.

• • •

When William H. McNeill was drafted into the U.S. Army in 1941, the Texas base he arrived at was undersupplied. For the first six weeks, each recruit had only one set of fatigues, producing a memorable stench. And although McNeill was training to become an antiaircraft artilleryman, the base had only a single nonfunctioning antiaircraft weapon for the entire battalion. McNeill's training officers struggled to fill the time on base with useful activities. They ordered the recruits to pick grass around the barracks by hand (one of the many supplies they lacked was a lawn mower). The officers also made the men in training march for hours in close formation. McNeill's first impression of these drills was "a more useless exercise would be hard to imagine." His view shifted, however, the longer they marched under the hot sun, their boots stomping dust and gravel, and their voices shouting *Hut! Hup! Hip! Four!* "Words are inadequate to describe the emotion aroused by the prolonged movement in unison that drilling involved," McNeill wrote in his 1995 book *Keeping Together in Time.* "A sense of pervasive well-being is what I recall; more specifically, a strange sense of personal enlargement; a sort of swelling out, becoming bigger than life."

Psychologists call this sense of empowerment through joint action *we-agency.* McNeill coined the term *muscular bonding* to describe how physical activities like marching and synchronized labor produce we-agency. When we move in unison, we become willing and able to give our all to a collective aim. After McNeill left the military and continued his career as a historian, he came to believe that the we-agency achieved through muscular bonding has been a source of military strength throughout history. The Aztecs, Spartans, and Zulus all used ritualized dancing to train young warriors, and European armies practiced close-order drills to build "a hunting band sociability" that would shore up soldiers' solidarity and commitment in battle.

McNeill's insight points to a second social function of synchronized movement. It isn't just about helping individuals build friendship networks. It's also about building a tribe that can defend its territory, pursue common goals, and face large threats together. Physician Joachim Richter and psychologist Roya Ostovar have speculated that early humans might have developed synchronized movement as a defense tactic, to "delude a predator by producing the impression of being a homogeneous enormous animal which would be too powerful to attack." This idea is not so farfetched. Many species deploy strategies of synchronized defense. Pilot whales and dolphins swim and surface in unison to intimidate outsiders. Yellow-rumped cacique birds protect their eggs from predators by forming a mob around the invader, diving at and pecking the predator until it flees. When muskoxen are surrounded by wolves, they pack themselves together tightly, horns facing out, to become a multiheaded beast, an impenetrable herd. Human groups moving in unison can produce a similarly daunting effect. In one psychology experiment, participants rated the formidability of groups of soldiers based only on the sounds of those groups approaching. In some of the audio recordings, the footsteps were synchronized; in others, the steps were not. When participants heard synchronized steps, they imagined the soldiers to be physically stronger and bigger. The synchronized groups were also perceived as more unified, no longer separate individuals but a single entity— a kind of superorganism—with an elevated capacity to fight.

Any group moving in unison is seen by others as united in purpose, connected by shared values, and acting as one. But as William H. McNeill observed while marching in basic training, this is not just an observer effect. Those in the group feel more powerful, too. When people move together, they view external threats as less fearsome and their opponents as less intimidating. This may be one reason why the Andaman Islanders performed dance rituals before a fight with an outside group. It's also part of why political and social movements organize marches. The collective movement not only demonstrates the strength of its coalition to outsiders but also bolsters the morale of its members. Studies of real-world marches and demonstrations confirm that participating in these events generates feelings of we-agency. Active participants—but not those who observe from the sidelines—describe feeling connected to the group and part of something bigger than themselves. Marching also makes participants more hopeful. After the event, they are more likely to agree that the world is becoming more just, that human nature is more good than evil, and that the problems they are protesting are solvable. Importantly, watching these events is not enough to produce these effects. You must join in.

Polina Davidenko was born in the Russian city of Omsk, in Siberia, and moved to the United States with her parents and sister when she was two years old. In 2008, when she was a freshman in high school, her grandmother Nina, still living in

Russia, was diagnosed with lymphoma. Neither Davidenko nor her mother could be with her, and the separation weighed on them both. Soon after the diagnosis, Davidenko's school hosted the American Cancer Society's Relay For Life fundraiser, where community members would walk the track around the high school's football field for twenty-four consecutive hours. As the American Cancer Society explains, "Cancer patients don't stop because they're tired, and for one night, neither do we." Davidenko decided to participate.

She recalls that the weather that day was perfect, sunny with no wind or rain. During the day, everyone was full of energy and the event felt like a party. Local bands performed on a stage, and the football field was transformed into a campsite, complete with food, tents, and foldout chairs. Davidenko's parents stopped by during the afternoon to walk a mile with her. After sunset, things got quieter. Walkers decorated white paper bags in tribute to survivors and loved ones lost to cancer, then lit candles in them to turn them into luminaries of hope. Davidenko made one for her grandmother and adorned it with flowers. As the walkers lapped the track in the darkness, they pointed out which luminaries they had made, and Davidenko got to share stories about her grandmother.

"Four A.M. is when the deeper conversations come out," Davidenko remembers. "When you're moving and talking, you feel more open to share than when sitting face-to-face. Your inhibitions are down, and you become more open to say things you otherwise wouldn't. Afterward, you trust people because they saw you in such a vulnerable state." Sometimes she walked in silence by herself, but even then, she says, "You still feel connected to something bigger than yourself. You're not just in your own thoughts. You can see the community on the field, playing games, crying, talking. You're a witness to all of that." She stopped counting at fifty laps and estimates that she walked twelve miles in the dark. "You notice the fatigue less because of the purpose. I couldn't walk fifty laps just for fun."

In the morning, local firefighters cooked a pancake breakfast and served sausages, bagels, and orange juice. Everyone ate together as the organizers made closing comments and thanked the walkers and volunteers. When Davidenko left, her sneakers were coated with the red dust of the football track. She remembers feeling proud of those sneakers and not wanting to wipe the dust off.

Psychologist Bronwyn Tarr told me, "We need things that help us connect with one another, that give us opportunities to forge collectivity." If we're lucky, we experience many such moments in everyday life, but it also helps to have special events that draw on the power of moving together. Researchers have studied the effects of participating in charity athletic events like the Relay For Life, and participants routinely describe feeling a collective strength, hope, and optimism. Organizations that host such events could choose any method of fundraising, from rummage sales to auctions, but none have the popular draw of 5Ks, half marathons, and physical challenges like Hustle Chicago, in which thousands of people climb the iconic John Hancock Tower's ninety-four stories to raise funds for the Respiratory Health Association. Threats on the scale of heart disease, cancer, AIDS, and social injustice can make us feel paralyzed, hopeless, or defeated. Athletic events that acknowledge these collective problems are opportunities to experience one of the antidotes to despair, we-agency. When we take our part in these collective endeavors, the physical movement uplifts us and the community inspires us. Winning the battle suddenly feels possible. It also reminds us that our struggles are shared by others. This was something Polina Davidenko told me. "When you're suffering from something, you forget that you're not alone in it. When you see people come together, it reminds you that you aren't alone."

Once a year, over a thousand people dance together on the deck of the USS *Midway*, an aircraft carrier docked in San Diego Harbor. Two hundred thousand sailors served on the USS *Midway* from 1945 to 1992, when it was deployed for both combat and humanitarian missions. Today the carrier hosts hundreds of military ceremonies and community events each year. One of these events is the annual Jazzercise Dance for Life fundraiser, which in one day raises over a hundred thousand dollars for breast cancer research and support. The event is advertised as a fight against breast cancer. Many of the dancers arrive in groups, wearing matching tank tops with slogans like "Strong alone. Unstoppable together." Instructors lead participants through dance routines to popular music, a thousand feet simultaneously striking the ship deck with every step. Aerial shots show a swarm of hot-pink-clad bodies moving in unison, suggesting a superorganism rather than a group of individuals. Through their synchronized steps and desire to come together, the dancers have become the impenetrable herd, a swarm defending its own, a throng of selves merged into a powerful *we*.

In March 2011, the Great East Japan Earthquake hit Iwanuma City hard. Half of the coastal city's land was submerged under tsunami waters, and 180 residents lost their lives. In the aftermath, 15 percent of the population developed symptoms of depression. As part of the city's recovery, public health officials developed programs to encourage residents to stay physically active. Those who increased their participation in group exercise were less likely to become depressed. Walking alone also had a protective effect, but the benefits of exercising in a group were stronger.

I thought about this in the fall of 2017, when I was in Houston to speak to the Texas Municipal League about resilience. The meeting, which brought together mayors, chiefs of police and fire chiefs, city council members and managers, and directors of public works, parks, and planning, took place on the heels of Hurricane Harvey, one of the worst natural disasters in Texas history. The George R. Brown Convention Center, where the event was taking place, had sheltered thousands of citizens whose homes had been damaged or destroyed by the hurricane.

The afternoon I arrived, I took a walk through downtown toward City Hall, where streets had flooded during the storm. As I walked back to my hotel, I heard music. I followed the sound to Discovery Green Park, where a free Zumba class was taking place across from the convention center. Dozens of dancers clapped and marched on stone tiles, led by a local instructor, Oscar Sajche, who demonstrated the moves from the bandstand. It was hot and humid, and I was already drenched with sweat from my walk. I had a bag full of groceries that needed to be refrigerated, but I hesitated only a moment before dropping my bag on a park chair and joining in.

We danced to all the usual rhythms of a Zumba class: salsa, reggaeton, cumbia, merengue, Pitbull. Some of the participants wore official Zumba tanks and tees, but many looked like me—inappropriately dressed for a workout, but unable to resist a dance party. Strangers smiled at me. People looked happy to be there. As we shimmied and stomped, it occurred to me that the very fact that we were dancing on this spot, so soon after a major natural disaster, was a sign of the city's resilience. Or maybe the dance party was something else: not so much proof of resilience as a source of resilience. Jacob Devaney, who rebuilt homes in New Orleans after Hurricane Katrina, remembers working from sunrise to late into the evenings, each day bringing more reminders and stories of what had been lost. Instead of going home to rest at the end of his shifts, Devaney went dancing in the New Orleans clubs. He attributes his ability to survive that period, without burning out or getting sick, to those early morning hours of collective joy.

When I tracked down the instructor of the outdoor Zumba class on Facebook, I discovered that Sajche had been teaching free community classes in Houston for over a decade. During the initial recovery from Hurricane Harvey, he had posted this message on Facebook: "Enjoy an awesome outdoor class with hundreds of Zumba warriors. We are Houston Strong and getting back on our feet." It struck me that offering that class was as much a model of civic engagement as the Municipal League event that had brought me to Houston. When I spoke to the public servants and officials the next day, I talked about purpose and social connection. I acknowledged the service project attendees had participated in the day before, sorting donations for a local food bank. And at the back of my mind, I thought, *Maybe I should have scrapped the speech and brought a great playlist.*

HUMAN BEINGS SYNCHRONIZE NATURALLY. Not just our movements, but every aspect of our physiology. When we feel connected to another person, our heartbeats, breathing, and even brain activity fall into step. Groups will often synchronize their movements and breathing even without explicit instructions to do so. People also synchronize with greater accuracy to another person's slightly irregular beat than to a perfect rhythm generated by a computer. It is as if our biology is tuned to recognize and respond to common humanity. For some people, reducing self-transcendence to a neurological quirk can be deflating. Yet I find myself captivated by the brain's eagerness to become part of something bigger. We are equipped with a perceptual system ready to abandon the tight confines of our usual sense of self. We were born with brains able to craft a sense of connection to others that is as visceral as the feedback coming from your own heart, lungs, and muscles. That is an astonishing thing, that humans can go about most of our lives, sensing and feeling ourselves as separate, but through one small action—coming together in movement—we dissolve the boundaries that divide us.

Cognitive scientist Mark Changizi uses the word *nature-harnessing* to describe any cultural invention that can "harness evolutionarily ancient brain mechanisms for a new purpose." Such inventions become widely popular because they tap into our core instincts. One of my motivations for exploring the research on collective joy was to better understand my love of group exercise. Now, as I reflect on what takes place in those classes, nature-harnessing seems exactly right. Any human who has ever danced around a fire or stomped their feet in some pre-battle ritual would know what to do in an aerobics class. Psychologist Bronwyn Tarr herself has said that if you're looking to experience collective joy, the most effective way would be "a massive Zumba class." Group exercise has managed to capitalize on many of the conditions that intensify the benefits of synchronized movement. For example, the more you get your heart rate up, the closer you feel to the people you move in unison with. Adding music has the same enhancing effect. Whether by design or accident, many exercise classes also take advantage of the "close clustering" phenomenon. Maintaining less personal space amplifies the social cohesion felt while moving in synchrony, perhaps because physical closeness further blurs the boundary between self and other. When we're close enough to smell one another, emotions become more contagious. Did you know that happy sweat has a different odor than ordinary sweat, and that when you smell someone else's happy sweat, it can elevate your mood, too? The scent of joy released through our pores appears to be culturally universal. Even when you don't speak the same language—such as when Bronwyn Tarr found herself dancing the carimbó on the island of Marajó—it is possible to be carried away by a collective happiness that you can literally breathe in.

The repetition of simple movements in popular group exercise formats further contributes to collective joy. Analyzing the dance rituals of the Andaman Islanders, A. R. Radcliffe-Brown could discern no obvious artistic value in the steps. "Their function seems to be to bring into activity as many of the muscles of the body as possible," he wrote. The uniformity and simplicity of movement ensured that the dancers experienced "a pleasure of self-surrender." Modern aerobics adopts the same strategy to produce a similarly ecstatic experience. When group exercise goes wrong, it's almost always because the movements are so complicated that the synchrony collapses and the individual falls out of step with the group.

Every decade, the fitness industry reinvents itself. But while the moves and music may change, and new tools—a step, weighted bars, stationary bikes—get added, those of us with decades of step-touches under our leotard belts can tell you that the core experience is the same. Whenever a new group exercise program takes off, it's often because it added synchrony to a typically unsynchronized physical activity, like boxing (Tae Bo), weight lifting (BodyPump), or cycling (SoulCycle). Remove the trappings of any fitness program at its cultural apex, and you'll find the same ingredients, the same collective joy. As long as our DNA compels us to connect with others, we will continue to seek out places where we can move and sweat together.

While most people find pleasure in synchronized movement, some people seem especially drawn to move in unison with others. One possible reason has to do with the link between collective joy and cooperation. It turns out that people who have a prosocial orientation to life—that is, they enjoy witnessing other people's happiness and are motivated to help others who are struggling—synchronize more easily with others. Something in their mindset or biology makes it easier to merge in collective action and lose themselves in the movement. Perhaps this is the final instinct group exercise harnesses: the desire to step outside oneself and to be of some use in the world. That this desire should express itself through synchronized step-touches, squats, and tap-backs may seem strange. Outsiders cannot understand the appeal; this is a joy for which spectatorship falls short. Like any nature-harnessing phenomenon, it doesn't make sense until you're in the middle of it. Then suddenly, endorphins flowing and heart pounding, you find it the most reasonable thing in the world. As historian William H. McNeill writes, "Euphoric response to keeping together in time is too deeply implanted in our genes to be exorcized for long. It remains the most powerful way to create and sustain a community that we have at our command."

Chapter 4

LET YOURSELF BE MOVED

A couple of years ago, I was backstage in a ballroom at the Hyatt Regency in downtown San Francisco, waiting to give the keynote at a conference for technology designers. The opening ceremony before my talk featured a group of Tibetan monks from the Drepung Loseling Monastery. The monks would be building a sand mandala, an intricate, labor-intensive art installation made from colored sands, in the hotel lobby over the three-day event. They were waiting with me backstage, lined up in their red robes, their arms resting under ceremonial gold wraps, hands clasped. As we waited, the sound system blasted music to draw attendees into the ballroom. When the Saint Motel song "Move" came on, I found myself nodding my head, captured by the infectious beat. Out of the corner of my eye, I noticed a brown leather slip-on loafer tapping the floor to the beat. The monk wearing the loafer caught me watching him and smiled.

In that moment, we were both driven by a powerful instinct: to move when we hear music. Musicologists call this urge *groove.* For most people, the impulse to synchronize our bodies to a beat is so strong, it takes effort to suppress it. It's an instinct that shows up early in life. Newborns out of the womb for only forty-eight hours can detect a regular beat. Infants rock their feet to the 4/4 meter of Mozart's *Eine kleine Nachtmusik* and smile while doing so. That these behaviors emerge before language, walking, or even crawling suggests that the ability to move to music—and enjoy it—is as innate a human capacity as you can find.

Indeed, the brain seems to be hardwired to hear music as an invitation to move. If you listen to music while lying motionless in a brain scanner, scientists will see your motor system light up. Music activates the so-called motor loop of the brain, including the supplementary motor area, which plans movement, the basal ganglia and the putamen, which coordinate movement, and the cerebellum, which controls the timing of movements. The stronger the musical beat or the more you like what you hear, the more feverishly these regions consume fuel. All of this happens even though you remain absolutely still. It's as if your brain can't hear music without recruiting the rest of the body. As neurologist Oliver Sacks wrote, "When listening to music, we listen with our muscles." One of the greatest pleasures in life is to give in to this impulse: to sing, to dance, to clap and stomp; to celebrate how notes and chords and lyrics reach inside you; and to surrender to their one command, *Let yourself be moved.*

• • •

On July 1, 1863, Private Robert Goldthwaite Carter, of Company H of the 22nd Massachusetts Infantry Regiment, was marching under the hot Pennsylvania sun. That day's twenty-mile trek would take Carter and his fellow soldiers on a path littered with dead horses, reminders of the Union cavalrymen killed in a battle the previous day. As Carter described in letters, many men suffered heatstroke, and as the afternoon sun peaked, "hundreds were falling exhausted by the roadside." Just when the regiment was on the verge of being defeated by fatigue, Carter heard bugles and drums in the distance. An unseen regiment marching on a parallel road had begun to play music.

> Every weary and footsore soldier, the halt, lame
> and chafed patriot, played out, exhausted and
> about to deposit his weary bones by the wayside,
> gathered inspiration from the sound, took the step,
> and with renewed courage plodded into camp. . . .
> Such was the power of music upon the drooping
> spirits of the rough, bronzed veterans of the
> gallant old Army of the Potomac.

Many endurance athletes have a similar story of being brought back to life by a well-timed song. Seventy-six-year-old Tucker Andersen, who has run the New York City Marathon almost every year since 1976, told *The New York Times* about a memorable race when music helped carry him to the finish line. He had just passed the twenty-mile mark, when many runners hit the wall. In the New York City Marathon, that "wall" coincides with crossing the Willis Avenue Bridge into the Bronx, where the throngs of cheering fans thin out. One year, as Andersen entered the Bronx, a teenager leaned out of an apartment window and, as if solely to give Andersen strength, held out a stereo blasting the theme song from *Rocky*.

The brain responds to music it enjoys with a powerful adrenaline, dopamine, and endorphin rush, all of which energize effort and alleviate pain. For this reason, musicologists describe music as *ergogenic*, or work-enhancing. Throughout history and across cultures, music has been used to make labor less difficult and more rewarding. The endorphins released by music not only make tasks easier but can also bond a group that works together. Bennett Konesni, who runs Duckback Farm in Belfast, Maine, has traveled the world studying work song traditions, spending time with musical fisherman in Ghana, dancing farmers in Tanzania, and singing shepherds in Mongolia. He and his Maine farm crew sometimes sing when they plant seeds and shuck garlic. "It's not like *The Sound of Music*," he told me. "You wait for your brain and body to need it." When Konesni launches into a work song, "Something changes pretty quick. I don't feel my muscles in the same way. The pain disappears, like I've taken Advil. I start to sweat more because I'm working harder, but I also find I'm working faster." As the physical discomfort recedes, pleasure takes over. "I start to feel this euphoria and timelessness, and I can't tell you how many minutes have gone by."

Thanks to its ergogenic effects, music can help people transcend their own apparent physical limitations. In one experiment, middle-aged patients with diabetes and high blood pressure listened to upbeat music as they completed a cardiovascular stress test. During the test, patients first walked and then ran on a treadmill for as long as they could, while the experimenter regularly ramped up both the speed and incline. Most people get winded by minute six and give up within eight. When accompanied by music, however, patients soldiered on for an average of fifty-one seconds longer. That's almost a full minute at their highest level of effort. A cardiovascular stress test is the gold standard for determining how strong your heart is and what you can endure. Music redefined what their hearts were capable of.

Many athletes have learned to exploit this benefit. In carefully controlled experiments, adding a soundtrack helps rowers, sprinters, and swimmers shave seconds off their times. Runners can tolerate extreme heat and humidity longer, and triathletes can push themselves farther before reaching exhaustion. Moving to music even leads athletes to consume less oxygen as they exert themselves, as if the song itself supplies some of the energy they need. Findings like this led the authors of a scientific review in the *Annals of Sports Medicine and Research* to conclude that music is a legal performance-enhancing drug.

In 2007, the U.S. governing body for running competitions barred the use of personal music players at official races. They claimed it was primarily for safety, but many assumed it was to prevent an unfair performance advantage from having the right playlist. This may be a legitimate concern. In 1998, Ethiopian athlete Haile Gebrselassie managed to convince event organizers to play the pop song "Scatman" over the sound system during the indoor 2,000-meter race. He had practiced to that song and knew it was the perfect track to synchronize his stride to. He ended up breaking the world record.

If music is a performance-enhancing drug, then Brunel University sports psychologist Costas Karageorghis is one of the world's leading suppliers. He works with Olympic, national, and collegiate athletes to create custom playlists for training and competitions. He's helped create the soundtracks for Run to the Beat, a music-driven half marathon, and O_2 Touch, a mixed-gender touch rugby program played to music. He's also responsible for shaping the algorithms that determine what songs you hear in the workout playlists of several prominent streaming services.

Karageorghis grew up in what he describes as a "poor but colorful enclave" of South London, in an apartment above a secondhand record store. Every morning he was jolted awake by the booming bass of the shop's subwoofer. After getting out of bed, he liked to look out his window at the people walking by. As soon as they came within earshot of the music—often the reggae sounds of Bob Marley or Desmond Dekker—they smiled and started to walk with a lilt in their step. It seemed to Karageorghis that adding a soundtrack to an ordinary stroll was transformative—creating what he calls "an auditory elation."

As a teenager, Karageorghis excelled in track and field, and one year he competed in junior track and field at the annual Grand Prix in London. He found himself in the warm-up area with legendary 400-meter hurdler Edwin Moses. Moses was listening to soul music on an early Sony Walkman. At the time, personal listening devices were rare, and Moses was the only athlete using music to prepare. Karageorghis remembers thinking how innovative this was, and how brilliant it was that Moses was able to create his own bubble to get into the right mindset.

Now personal music players are ubiquitous, and Karageorghis is the one helping athletes choose the songs they listen to. He starts by trying to figure out each athlete's musical tastes. What are their favorite songs? Who are their favorite artists? He'll review their music library track by track, asking them to explain why they like specific songs. He'll put them on a treadmill to find out which tracks increase their speed. He'll test their hand-grip strength to discover if a song boosts their ability to push through fatigue. Karageorghis is looking for a power song—one that resonates so strongly that it alters the athlete's mood and physiology. He can often tell right away when he's hit on an effective track. "You immediately observe a rhythm response," he says. The athlete starts bobbing his head or tapping her toes. There are also the telltale signs of physiological arousal, such as dilated pupils and piloerection, when the hair on your skin stands on end. This is how Karageorghis knows the song is triggering an adrenaline rush.

Power songs tend to share certain qualities that make them stimulating: a strong beat, an energetic feel, and a tempo of around 120 to 140 beats per minute, which seems to be a universally preferred cadence for human movement. Power songs also have strong "extramusical" associations: the positive emotions, images, and meaning the song triggers in the listener. These associations can be based on the lyrics, the performers, one's own personal memories, or pop culture—for example, if a song was in the soundtrack to a film or if it served as an official song for a major sporting event.

Of all a song's qualities, lyrics are the most important for pushing us to work harder and for reducing fatigue, pain, and perceived effort. If you look at popular workout playlists, you'll see song after song with lyrics that emphasize qualities like perseverance and determination. This is one reason Eminem's "Till I Collapse" remains the most popular workout song of all time. Effective power songs often have lyrics that relate to physical activity itself, with words like *work, go,* or *run.* After Karageorghis mentioned this, I looked through my music library and realized he was right—some of my own power songs are

"Let's Go" by Travis Barker, "Work" by Stella Mwangi, and "Move (Keep Walkin')" by TobyMac.

Many athletes respond to music that inspires heroic imagery. One of Karageorghis's studies found that listening to "Eye of the Tiger" by Survivor (the theme song to *Rocky III*) helped participants work harder and enjoy themselves more during a strength challenge performed to exhaustion. No doubt part of the song's power lies in its association with a fighter who won't quit and its lyrics about rising to a challenge. Recordings of brain activity revealed that the song distracted participants from their effort, allowing them to push past the first signs of discomfort that typically make us quit before we reach our actual physical limits.

I can still remember the first time I heard what would become one of my go-to power songs. I was in an indoor cycling class when "Warrior" by Australian pop singer Havana Brown came on. The track has a hard-driving beat and a female vocalist singing about dancing to the beat of a drum, backed by male voices shouting what sounds like "Go! Go! Go!" By the time we got to the first chorus, it was like the song had entered my body. I felt a wildness I associate with intoxication or infatuation. It was like I had discovered an unknown reserve of energy, and once I was plugged into that reserve, the energy surged through my blood, helping me push the pedals faster and with more force. I turned the resistance wheel up not because the instructor told us to, but because I wanted to feel the pedals push back. I wanted to sense my own power and strength as I overcame the resistance. The best way I can describe it is that the song set my brain on fire. It kindled all the right neurons, triggering a primal response that tapped into my very identity; it wasn't lost on me that the Gaelic meaning of my name, Kelly, is "warrior."

Karageorghis's research shows that at moderate levels of

intensity, music reduces perceived effort, making the work feel easier and more enjoyable. But at higher intensities, when you're struggling to continue, it no longer reduces that perceived effort. Instead, it colors your interpretation of what you're feeling, adding a positive meaning to the physical discomfort. When you hear Eminem rap about finding your inner strength or Beyoncé tell you that a winner don't quit on themselves, the sweat, the fatigue, the burning in your lungs—they all become evidence of your determination, fortitude, and stamina. In this way, the right playlist can transform your experience of exercise. In a study at the University of Otago in New Zealand, researchers asked women to say out loud what they were thinking as they ran on a treadmill. The women's minds often returned to sensations of effort. For one woman, breathing harder and sweating might be interpreted as meaning *I am getting stronger* or *I am doing something good for my body*. To another woman, the same sensations might lead to thoughts of *I am too out of shape to do this*. These interpretations in turn predicted how much the women enjoyed working out. When they took a positive view of the sensations of effort, they felt much more pleasure. This was most true when they reached what's called the ventilatory threshold, the point at which you have to breathe harder to fuel your heart. Music is one way to shape the meaning of what you feel when you work hard. When you choose songs that inspire you, every burst of effort can also empower the story you want to tell about who you are and who you are becoming.

When Amara MacPhee woke up from surgery in the cardiothoracic unit at NewYork-Presbyterian/Weill Cornell Medical

Center, the pain was excruciating. There were tubes running in and out of her body and machines beeping. She couldn't sit upright. MacPhee remembers being utterly overwhelmed and thinking, *This is going to be way harder than I thought it would be.*

A month earlier, forty-year-old MacPhee had been in the best shape of her life, thanks to the classes she was taking at 305 Fitness in New York City's West Village. MacPhee loved the high-energy music, the live DJ, and the studio's disco lights. She also relished the community spirit. She liked that when the class made it through the hardest part of the workout—a nonstop cardio section called the sprint—the instructor would say, "High-five your neighbor, tell them congrats!"

One Saturday morning in September 2016, MacPhee found herself coughing through class. She thought maybe it was allergies. The following Tuesday, she had an even harder time breathing in class and had to take more water breaks than usual. *Maybe I'm getting bronchitis*, she thought. She went to her doctor, assuming she'd get a prescription for antibiotics and be better in a week. Instead, her doctor kept her stethoscope over MacPhee's lower left side for what felt like a long time. "I want to send you for a chest X-ray," she said. When the results came back, MacPhee's doctor traced the image with a pencil, saying, "This is your heart. These are your lungs." Then she circled a big gray spot between MacPhee's left lung and her rib cage. "I need to send you to the hospital for a CAT scan."

The scan revealed a mass the size of a grapefruit. MacPhee had a benign thymoma, a rare growth that starts in the cells of the thymus, an immune organ behind the sternum. The pressure on her left lung had been making it hard to breathe. MacPhee's tumor was not cancerous, but she would need to undergo open heart surgery to remove it.

The first time she tried to get out of bed after the surgery, her legs felt like rubber. She had to lean to the side because it hurt too much to stand up straight. When her physical therapist told her it was time to try walking, she managed to stagger down the hall to the nurses' station and back to her room. "It seemed like a never-ending hallway," MacPhee remembers. "I felt like I had run a marathon."

A few days later, her husband arrived at the hospital with a surprise. "Listen to this, I promise, you'll like it," he told her. She put in an earbud and heard a song she recognized as a 305 Fitness warm-up track. "Sadie sent it for you!" her husband said. One of MacPhee's instructors had put together a playlist of her favorite tracks from class. She told her husband she wanted to try walking again.

MacPhee's husband helped her out of bed. She was still in her hospital gown, robe, and socks with skids on the bottom. With one hand, she dragged the rolling stand that held her IV drip. With her other hand, she held on to her husband for support. She kept one earbud in, the other out so she could hear her husband encouraging her. The hallway was still cold and depressing, but the playlist—including Rihanna's "We Found Love" and RuPaul's "Sissy That Walk"—transported her. They were her power songs. MacPhee felt like she was in class instead of the hospital. "It made me feel like I was surrounded by people cheering me on. It made me feel, *You can do this.*"

Three weeks after surgery, MacPhee posted a quote from Martin Luther King Jr. on Instagram: "If you can't fly, run. If you can't run, walk. If you can't walk, crawl. But by all means, keep moving." Seven weeks after surgery, she made it back to 305 Fitness. It was Thanksgiving weekend, and she was grateful to be moving again. As she celebrated with the community that had helped her pull through, it was all she could do to hold back the tears. At the end of class, her instructor Sadie announced, "I just want to say a special shout-out—Amara had some major surgery, and we missed her."

In our conversations, MacPhee referred to 305 Fitness as her Fit Fam, a phrase that brought my thoughts back to collective joy, and how moving together can forge strong bonds. Music can enhance these effects, whether it's accompanying the synchronized step-touches in a group exercise class or the muscular bonding of athletes in training. When I asked sports psychologist Costas Karageorghis if he had a favorite story from his career, he surprised me with a tale not about the power of music to make Olympians run faster, but its ability to bring people together. In 1997, the collegiate track and field club that Karageorghis managed was fraught with team conflict. Some of the athletes were avoiding each other on the bus and in hotels, and the discord was bringing down the entire team. Karageorghis had the idea to create a motivational video that highlighted the athletes who were not getting along. He combined footage of them in races, including cooperating in relays, and set it to the song "We Are Family" by Sister Sledge. Right before each meet, Karageorghis would play the highlight video for everyone. The team came together, and that year—for the first and only time in the club's history—they defeated their rival in the national championship.

This could have been just another example of Karageorghis motivating his athletes with music, but there was more to the story that he was eager to share. One member of that year's team worked as a DJ at the student union bar, where Karageorghis would sometimes stop for a drink at the end of his day. Whenever the DJ saw him there, he would play "We Are Family." Karageorghis's athletes would take the drink out of his hand and force him onto the dance floor. "I felt at one with the athletes," he remembers, and twenty years later, the song brings back all those feelings of belonging. A few days after he told me this story, Karageorghis sent me a photo of a red T-shirt bearing the Brunel University logo and the words *We Are Family*. He had made the T-shirts for the track and field team back in 1997, and he had held on to his all these years.

• • •

At the 2017 annual Stanford Dance Marathon, members of the Stanford community danced for twenty-four hours to raise over a hundred thousand dollars for the families and patients at the Lucile Packard Children's Hospital. The marathon took place on the basketball court of the athletic center, which had been decorated with balloons and student-made banners. Many participants accessorized their official Dance Marathon T-shirts with tutus and face glitter. The Stanford mascot, a nine-foot-tall dancing redwood tree, stopped by with the university cheerleaders to support the dancers. A steady stream of deliveries from a local pizza joint, Mexican grill, and bagel shop made sure everyone was fed.

The organizers had arranged for entertainment throughout the event to keep the marathoners engaged. Alongside a roster of live DJs, musical acts, and dance performances, I was scheduled to lead a one-hour dance party with easy-to-follow choreography and a playlist that would keep people moving and smiling. The dancers filled the court at least ten rows back. With no stage, only the first couple of rows could see me, and without a microphone, I couldn't verbally cue the moves. I had to trust that the dance steps would trickle back, and for the most part, they did.

As the big finale, I had chosen "You Can't Stop the Beat" from the film version of the Broadway musical *Hairspray*. Reviewers called the song jubilant, joyous, and contagiously elating— exactly how I feel when dancing to it. The piece is marked by fast percussion, cheerful trumpets that add a syncopated beat, and an upward melodic motion. The singers' perfectly harmonized voices praise not only the pleasures of shaking and shimmying on a Saturday night, but also the values of self-acceptance, equality, and social progress. I hoped that even if the marathon dancers didn't know the song, they would connect to its infectious energy. And to my delight, that's exactly what happened. The whole group caught on to the steps quickly, and they moved in unison, clapping and sashaying as if they had rehearsed the routine for hours. Many of the dancers knew the words, and I watched as students in the front row turned to their friends, smiling as they sang along. Later, an event organizer would tell me it was one of the most talked-about highlights of the marathon.

In a video of us dancing to the song, there is a moment about halfway through that captures the energy that spread through the sea of dancers. A young man in the very back is grinning and moving with the group, but not quite dancing full-out. Then as the song approaches the second chorus, he leans back, throws his head and arms to the sky, and starts pumping his hands in the air, all while belting out the lyrics. It was an eruption of happiness, as if the music had entered his body and filled him with a joy that had to be expressed.

Watch the official music video to the 2013 song "Happy" by Pharrell Williams, and you'll see people lip-synching, strutting, clapping, snapping, jumping, bouncing, swaying, and spinning. The song was a number one hit in twenty-four countries, and the video—which *Fast Company* called "as cheering as an opiate and just as addictive"—played a major role. "Happy" is essentially an instructional video for finding joy by moving in happy ways to happy music. This truly is one of the greatest thrills of movement: When a piece of music that *sounds* happy makes us *feel* happy, so much so that we must move in ways that *express* happiness—a positive feedback loop that accelerates and amplifies the joyous feelings induced by the song.

The similarities between happy music and joyful movement are striking. Songs that people describe as sounding happy tend to be up-tempo, higher-pitched, relatively loud, in a major key, and with a strong beat. Movements that people describe as looking happy share these qualities. Joyful movements are fast, big, and vertical. Happiness bounces, leaps, and jumps. It is upward-facing and expansive. A joyful body reaches out, looks to the sky, and takes up space. In one study, psychologists and musicologists at Dartmouth College created a computer program that could produce both piano melodies and animations of a bouncing ball with eyes. Users were instructed to create either songs or animations that depicted different emotions. When participants tried to express joy, their melodies sounded like their animations moved. A happy piano melody and a happy bouncing ball both had a regular, relatively fast beat. Both "faced up" through a higher pitch or eyes gazing upward. Participants also expressed happiness through increasingly larger steps in pitch or height—like a child on a trampoline, gleefully jumping higher and higher, or ravers bouncing up and down, gaining height and energy as the electronic dance music builds to a big break. Moving in this way can induce joy. In a series of experiments conducted around the world, anthropologists asked people of all ages to perform specific physical actions and report how they felt. Different movements reliably produced distinct emotions, including anger, sadness, and happiness. One movement pattern was more effective than any other at invoking a strong emotion. It was the signature expression of joy: a full-body jumping gesture, arms stretched overhead, chest open, and gaze lifted, as if you had just thrown confetti into the air.

In the study led by Dartmouth College researchers, members of an isolated village in Cambodia produced "happy" songs and "happy" animations similar to those of students in the United States, suggesting something universal about how joy sounds and moves. Many traditional dances from around the world and the music that accompanies them share these joyful qualities. Bhangra ("intoxicated with joy"), a dance from the Punjab region of India, is characterized by bouncing, clapping, and upward arm gestures, along with bold jumps and kicks. The Israeli folk song "Hava Nagila" ("Let Us Have Joy") is commonly accompanied by a dance of light and nimble leaps, arms stretched out or lifted overhead, often done in a circle, the dancers clapping and singing together. These dances capture something authentic about what happiness feels like and how we show it. Many dance traditions, and the music that accompanies them, persist not only because of their cultural legacy but also because they are effective vehicles for expressing joy. As British anthropologist A. R. Radcliffe-Brown observed in 1922, "The individual shouts and jumps for joy; the society turns the jump into a dance, the shout into a song."

When I first viewed a composite video of the bouncing ball animations intended to express happiness, I was reminded of the jumping dance of the Maasai warriors in Kenya. In this ritual, young men form a circle and, one or two at a time, come to the center to show off their jumps. They jump vertically, in one spot, with as much grace and height as they can. The other men sing as they watch, raising the pitch and volume of their voices to match the height of the dancers' jumps. The ritual is meant to be a competition, but sometimes the elation of the movement at the center of the circle is so contagious, the entire group forgets the rivalry and erupts into synchronized singing and jumping. When you watch such a moment, you can't help but think, *This is what joy looks like.*

I met Miriam, a seventy-five-year-old retired computer specialist and grandmother of nine, in a dance class at the Juilliard School at Lincoln Center in New York City. Like most of the attendees at this class, Miriam has Parkinson's disease. She was diagnosed in September 2015, but looking back, she realizes she had symptoms the previous spring. On a walking tour in the Chelsea neighborhood of Manhattan, she hadn't been able to keep up with the group. At the time she told herself it was because she was tired and it was warmer than she had expected. But now she realizes it was bradykinesia, the physical slowness that is one of the earliest signs of Parkinson's disease. When she visited her daughter a few months later, her daughter said, "What happened to you, Mom? You look like you aged ten years since I saw you."

Miriam's doctor told her that movement was the best thing she could do to delay the progression of the disease. He encouraged her to exercise for two hours a day. "It doesn't matter what kind," he said, "as long as you move." Miriam started taking classes at the YMCA. During one calisthenics session, the instructor left the room to get help with a broken air-conditioning system. She kept the music on in the background and encouraged the students to continue while she stepped out. When the Broadway classic "Don't Cry for Me Argentina," came on, Miriam began to sing along. To her surprise, singing made the movement easier. "I wasn't thinking, *Now I have to move my foot to the side*," she told me. "I just did it."

When she heard about the Dance for PD program at a health fair, she registered the next day. From the moment the pianist played a song from *West Side Story*, she knew she was going to love it. During class, she feels a lightness and ease in her body. She is graceful, not clumsy; elegant, not encumbered. Her body responds to the music in a way that makes her feel confident, less cautious and afraid. "The music reaches me," she says.

I attend one of the Dance for PD classes at Juilliard on a beautiful afternoon in June. Sunlight streams into the studio through a wall of windows. The dance floor, a traditional smooth black marley, has been staged with four concentric circles of plastic chairs. A piano stands in the corner. As participants arrive, they leave walkers and canes under the ballet bars or roll their wheelchairs into an opening in one of the circles. Many remove their shoes so they can dance barefoot or in socks. Class begins with a dramatic piano chord.

The instructor, Julie Worden, is a professional dancer who performed with the Mark Morris Dance Group for eighteen years. Worden leads us through a warm-up that the dance company uses to get rid of pre-performance jitters. We make faces, stretching the muscles of our cheeks, mouth, foreheads, and eyes. We make noises. It loosens us up. Still seated, we sing "Amazing Grace," but not with words—just sounds. We hum and *aaahhhh* the melody. "Let the music move through you," Worden tells us.

We learn modified choreography to a celebrated Mark Morris routine. Worden explains the nuances of each section, emphasizing the expressivity inspired by the music and emotion. We may be seated in chairs, stretching a foot to the left, instead of leaping, toes pointed, across a stage. But there is no implication that what we are doing is any less artistic, intentional, or beautiful. Worden insists we reach to the very tip of our fingers, like a trained dancer's elegant port de bras. After the warm-up, those who can, stand. We cha-cha around our chairs, while the pianist changes the tempo. "Follow the music!" Worden encourages. We listen and let the music guide us. Our steps become quick, then slower. Our hips swing fast and playfully, then languorously, sensually.

Finally assistants help us drag the chairs to the circumference of the room, and we begin to move across the floor. We walk, swinging our arms and taking big steps. I am spellbound by the difference in the quality of movement happening in the room at this point compared to when people first arrived. Many of the dancers had struggled just to get settled in their chairs before class began. That cautious shuffling is now gone, replaced by a liberated stride. It is as if before the first piano chord, their bodies had been windup toys insufficiently keyed. Now their springs were fully tightened, their bodies propelled forward by an energy ready to be released.

For our last dance, we perform a grand right and left—two

large circles moving in opposite directions. We greet each person we pass with a handshake and a smile. Pragmatics trump aesthetics here. The flow of the circles slows down as some exchanges take more time. Detours are arranged to include dancers unable to move their wheelchairs. One woman's assistant moves her arm for her, to allow her to shake each hand and make eye contact with each passing dancer. As we greet one another, it feels as if the entire class has been a prelude to this moment.

Months after I participated in the Dance for PD class, as I was poring over the neuroscience of music, I found myself thinking about that grand right and left—how we greeted one another with handshakes and smiles. Movement is necessary for the most basic forms of self-expression, including speech, facial expressions, and gestures. The body is how we translate what is happening inside us—thoughts, feelings, desires—into something observable that other people can understand.

Slowed walking and tremors are the most visible and familiar symptoms of Parkinson's disease. But there are also more subtle changes, including how the disease interferes with the ability to express emotions. A facial expression is a physical action that, like walking or running, depends on the coordination of many muscles. A genuine smile recruits at least a dozen muscles to lift the corners of your mouth, crinkle your eyes, and raise your cheeks. These actions, like other movements, are impaired in Parkinson's disease, creating a symptom called *facial masking*. It's as if the disease puts a plaster of Paris mask on the individual, concealing their true feelings and giving the impression of a mild, unchanging dissatisfaction. The mask is often misread as apathy or confusion, leading others to view individuals with Parkinson's as less intelligent, happy, and appealing as social partners.

All of us rely on the constant waltz of expressions across our faces to convey our insides to the outside world. When Parkinson's paralyzes this dance, the absence of movement becomes isolating. But just as music can help individuals with Parkinson's walk with greater ease, it can also reawaken the muscles that let us express and connect. Music triggers spontaneous facial expressions of emotion. When you listen to joyful music, the zygomaticus major—the muscle that draws the corner of your lips toward your cheekbone when you smile—contracts reflexively, similar to when a physician taps your kneecap to make your leg swing.

This spontaneous expression occurs in part because the emotion conveyed by music is contagious. Music activates the brain's mirror neuron system, which helps us recognize and understand what others are thinking and feeling. Mirror neurons sense and encode the emotions conveyed by sounds, voice, body language, and gesture. These neurons also prime the unconscious mimicry we engage in when we want to connect with others. Smiling when someone smiles at you. Allowing another person's laughter to elicit genuine laughter in you. Returning the grasp of a firm handshake or the embrace of a warm hug. Like the expression of emotion, spontaneous mimicry is impaired by Parkinson's disease, creating yet another barrier to social connection. Music and dance can help break through this barrier. One 2011 study, conducted in Freiburg, Germany, found that weekly dance classes modeled on the Dance for PD program softened facial masking and increased emotion expression.

The class I attended at Juilliard ended in a circle, with all of us holding hands. Our instructor explained that we would close by "passing our joy." One at a time, each dancer would physically express delight in movements, gestures, facial expressions, or sounds, then turn to the person to their right and invite them to express themselves next. As our joy made its way around the room, we smiled, squealed, blew kisses, raised our arms, lifted our heads, clapped our hands, and shimmied our shoulders. When it was my turn, I wagged my tail like a puppy. We laughed with one another. There was a palpable sense of approval and acceptance as each dancer made their offering. After the delight had gone around the entire group, we showed our gratitude and respect with a bow to the dancer on our right.

That afternoon, the ability to not just *feel* joy but *show* joy and share it with others was music's most profound gift. Music was the energizing force that allowed us to feel, express, and connect. The piano chords ignited neurons that greased the nervous system and allowed dormant muscle fibers to fire. Physical stuckness softened, then stretched into the embodiment of joy—sometimes in sweeping gestures, face lifting, arms raised to the sky, and sometimes in more subtle movements, the corners of the lips reaching upward.

MY LOVE OF DANCE COMES from my mother's side of the family. My grandfather served in World War II, stationed first in France, then Germany. He was in Czechoslovakia, waiting to be shipped to Japan, when the war ended. After he returned home, he contemplated joining the seminary to become a priest. Instead, he went to work for the U.S. Postal Service, riding the Reading Railroad nightly between Philadelphia and New York City to transport mail. He always said his decision came down to one thing: He didn't want to give up dancing to the big band music of Tommy and Jimmy Dorsey.

In December 1946, he met my grandmother at Wagner's Ballroom in Philadelphia. He noticed her standing alone and told her where she should stand so that she would be asked to dance. She took his advice and jitterbugged with many returning soldiers that night. My grandfather waited until the last song, a fox-trot to Irving Berlin's "Always," to invite her to dance. Then he walked her to the Broad Street subway and asked if he could meet her at the ballroom the following weekend.

After they married, one of the highlights of their life together was the annual dinner-dance for employees of the Philadelphia post office. My grandfather loved to tell the story of how in 1960, he was the only employee brave enough to try the hot new dance, Chubby Checker's "The Twist." While raising my mother and uncle, he worked two shifts: sorting mail for the post office from four P.M. to midnight, then delivering newspapers from one to five in the morning. Before he left for his first shift, he would lie on his back on the floor in the living room, his head close to the stereo, listening to his favorite records. My mother, who would often arrive home from school to find him on the floor, thought he was napping. When she was older, he told her it had been his way of dealing with chronic headaches. The music made the pain recede.

When my grandfather retired, my grandparents left their Northeast Philadelphia row house for a ranch home in Leisuretowne, New Jersey, and he became the chairman of the retirement community's monthly ballroom dances. He selected the music, while my grandmother scoured thrift shops for a new gown to wear to each dance. My grandfather chaired those dances for years, until complications from a hip replacement left my grandmother unable to move on her own.

She died in 2007, and my grandfather's heart weakened. Walking became difficult. He spent most of the day at home, sitting in the same chair. One day he stepped outside to get the mail, slipped, and lay on the ground for hours before a neighbor found him. Each Sunday when he attended mass, the walk from pew to priest weighed on his mind throughout the service. He was worried he would fall on the way to receiving communion. Three times he was taken by ambulance to the hospital with heart and kidney failure. Each time our family was told that he would not survive, and my mother brought a priest to the hospital to give him last rites. But his heart refused to give out for good. "God will take me when he wants me," he would say.

Two weeks after his third hospital stay, my mother learned that a Philadelphia string band was going to perform at the retirement community. She asked my grandfather if he wanted to go, and he said yes. The event was in same room as the ballroom dances he had chaired. He insisted on attending with his walker, not his wheelchair. My mother was afraid he would suffer another heart failure just trying to get to their seats.

The string band played many tunes he knew, and during some songs, the band asked the audience to sing along. My mother noticed a change in her father's face. "In those last years, he never said he was in pain," she remembers. "But his face was always troubled." Now the worried look was gone. When the band started strumming a popular parade song, my grandfather rose from his chair and, to my mother's utter astonishment, stepped into the aisle without his walker. He threw his hands in the air and began doing the Mummers' Strut. Other seniors joined him, and soon the aisle was filled, my grandfather leading them all in the dance. My mother couldn't believe what she was seeing. "I was shaking. My heart was pounding. He was so weak and so frail," she recalls. "I was sure he was going to pass out and fall. I thought I was going to have to pick him up off the floor." When the song was over, my grandfather took his seat next to my mother, smiling. He didn't say anything, just enjoyed the rest of the show. He lived another few months but never danced again.

Years later, my mother and I still wonder about that moment. I wasn't there, but I like to imagine it. I ask her more details. What was the song? What did he look like? And I ask her over and over, "What do you think happened?" "What do I think happened?" she repeats, sounding just as puzzled every time. "I don't know." I can hear the amazement in her voice as she relives the shock of the moment. "I think the music snapped something in him," she decides. "For that one moment, he wasn't afraid."

The power of music to move us can seem like magic. It makes miracles happen. In testimony to the U.S. Senate Special Committee on Aging in August 1991, neurologist Oliver Sacks told the story of a woman whose leg was completely paralyzed after a complex bone fracture. The doctors could find no evidence of any communication between her leg muscles and spinal cord. Everything suggested that her brain was no longer able to feel or control her leg. And yet her foot would tap spontaneously to the sound of an Irish jig. The doctors were able to exploit this bizarre exception, and through music therapy, she learned to walk and even dance again.

Music can reach inside you, tap into your most primal self. As a young Virginia Woolf wrote in her journal in 1903, "It stirs some barbaric instinct—lulled asleep in our sober lives—you forget centuries of civilization in a second, and yield to that strange passion which sends you madly whirling round the room." Even if the body cannot comply, the feeling of being moved persists. In a study of women living with chronic debilitating pain, one woman described the therapeutic effects of music. "Even when I'm just listening, doing nothing but lying there on the couch listening to music, there will be some part of my body that's moving in some way. I can feel my muscles shifting around in my body. . . . it feels like the music comes through my body. . . . like I'm doing what the musicians are doing. I can feel in my body what it feels like to blow that flute to make that sound."

Music can also help us access memories. We hear a song and remember a time, a place, a feeling. One woman reminisced to me about learning to ski at age sixteen, the year she discovered the Beatles. She remembers swinging downhill, humming tracks from *Sgt. Pepper's Lonely Hearts Club Band*. To this day, those songs bring her back to that time in her life, to the joy of mastering tight turns on the slope. Josh White, an Elvis impersonator who visits long-term senior care facilities around the United States, has seen people in noncommunicative, even comatose states reanimate when they hear a specific song. Their eyes open and light up. Sometimes they start singing along. "Even if the brain is literally dissolving," he told me, "they can still hang on to memories of their favorite music."

When you let yourself be moved by music, you lay down tracks in your nervous system, pathways for joy to traverse when you hear that song again. I know that when I choose to dance today, I am building muscle memories of joy, giving my future self more songs to be moved by. Bernie Salazar, a thirty-nine-year-old dad living in Chicago, told me about the dance parties he has with his daughter. Her favorite songs are "Happy" by Pharrell Williams and "Shake It Off" from the movie *Sing*. "There's a light that shines above her and us—we're in our own little joy force field. No disco ball can outshine what goes on in our living room," he says. "I've run three marathons and four half marathons, but I've never felt so high as losing myself in movement with my kid." His daughter has reached the age when she will bring her play phone to Salazar and say, "More more more," asking him to play music and dance with her. Most recently, she made that request in Target. "I don't care if she wants to dance in a grocery store, I'm going to break it down right there," he told me. Those are the moments he knows he will remember, the memories he wants to collect. "The old Bernie would have been, 'You can't do this, what are other people going to think?' They're going to forget about it, and that time will be lost if you don't."

According to my mother, my grandparents often sang the chorus of "Always," the song they first danced to in 1946, to each other. It was a ritual, a way of remembering. I never witnessed this. While writing this chapter, I looked up the song, found a Frank Sinatra recording from 1947, and listened to it late at night. As I heard the lyrics for the first time, I thought, *No wonder they got married.* How could you hold someone in your arms and dance to that song and not fall in love? Irving Berlin wrote it in 1925 as a wedding gift to his wife. In the lyrics, he promises to be there for her, not just for a day or year, but for always. When my grandparents danced for the first time, they had no way of knowing they were listening to the rest of their love story.

I was so moved by the song, I woke my husband up and dragged him out of bed. We danced barefoot, my head on his chest, laying down a new memory and feeling connected to the past.

Chapter 5

OVERCOMING OBSTACLES

Cathy Merrifield stood on the edge of the twelve-foot-high platform, staring into a pit of muddy water. It was her first Tough Mudder obstacle course, and the forty-four-year-old mother of four was waiting for her turn to jump. Her shoes were duct-taped to her feet to make sure they wouldn't come off. Safety divers were on standby, and friends and strangers who had already taken the plunge were cheering her on. Her boyfriend was standing on the sidelines, camera aimed to capture her jump. She agreed to go with a friend on the count of three, but when *three* came, her feet stayed firmly planted. As she looked down, the platform seemed much higher than it had from the ground. Her stomach was in knots, and she realized she was holding her breath. This was the obstacle she had been dreading the most, and she didn't know if she could do it.

When Merrifield was eight years old, her mother sent her to swim lessons at the local YMCA. One day the kids lined up to practice jumping off the high dive. When it was Merrifield's turn, she froze on the diving board, too scared to jump. She turned to climb back down, but as she remembers it, the swim instructor came up the ladder, blocked her exit, and threatened to push her off the diving board. With no other option, she jumped, and as she plunged under the surface, water rushed into her airway. Although that swim lesson was almost forty years ago, Merrifield easily recalls her terror. "I remember the feeling of *I have to do this, there's not going to be a choice. I can't go back down the ladder.* That dread of *I'm going to have to do this even though I don't want to.*" Now, standing on the Tough Mudder platform, she had an opportunity to rewrite the ending. This time, the decision of whether to jump or not would be hers alone. She held her nose, closed her eyes, and leapt.

So much of the language we use to describe courage relies on metaphors of the body. We overcome obstacles, break through barriers, and walk through fire. We carry burdens, reach out for help, and lift one another up. This is how we as humans talk about bravery and resilience. When we are faced with adversity or doubting our own strength, it can help to feel these actions in our bodies. Sometimes we need to climb an actual hill, pull ourselves up, or work together to shoulder a heavy load to know that these traits are a part of us. The mind instinctively makes sense out of physical actions. When you embrace the metaphorical meaning of movements, you can literally sense the strength that is in you and the support that is available to you.

Human beings are also storytellers, and the stories we choose to tell shape how we think about ourselves and the world. One of the most powerful ways that movement can affect us is through its ability to change our most deeply held stories. Whether it's by plunging into a pool of muddy water, learning how to hold a headstand, or lifting more weight than you ever thought possible, physical accomplishments can change how you think about yourself and what you are capable of. Do not underestimate how significant such a breakthrough can be. When Araliya Ming Senerat was in her early twenties, she was depressed, living in a city far away from her family and friends, and unhappy at work. She made a plan to take her own life. The day she intended to go through with it, she went to the gym for one last workout. She deadlifted 185 pounds, a personal best. When she put the bar down, she realized that she didn't want to die. Instead, she remembers, "I wanted to see how strong I could become." Five years later, she can now deadlift 300 pounds.

• • •

The first time I heard of Tough Mudder—a ten-mile obstacle course described as the "toughest event on the planet"—was from a psychology student who raved about how fun it was. He offered me a discount code if I wanted to try it myself. I looked the event up online, saw photos of obstacles like Boa Constrictor, Trench Warfare, and Ladder to Hell, and thought, *No thanks, no way, not in a million years.* My first impression of Tough Mudder, with its simulated tear gas tunnels and slides set on fire, was that it was a jungle gym for masochists looking to prove their toughness. This is not an uncommon take on the event; journalist Lizzie Widdicombe likened it to a rite of passage in which boys "are initiated into manhood if they can keep their hands in a glove filled with stinging ants for several minutes without screaming." But as I read accounts and talked to people who had completed the course, I heard stories of discovery, empowerment, and even redemption. People were overcoming obstacles in ways that became self-defining moments.

To better understand what was happening on the course, I reached out to Nolan Kombol, the company's lead obstacle designer. Kombol grew up on a farm near Enumclaw, Washington, where he was routinely shocked by cattle fences—an experience that helped Kombol contribute to the design of the Tough Mudder's most infamous obstacle, Electroshock Therapy, using electrified cattle fence wires. Kombol explained that when the design team sits down to dream up new obstacles, they don't ask, "How can we hurt people?" Their goal is to create a story people will want to tell afterward. The surface story may be "I ran through electricity," but the deeper story is "I did something I never thought I could do."

Obstacle designers target common phobias, like confined spaces, contamination, heights, or the dark. The idea is to provoke just enough fear that the obstacle requires courage to complete. One of the most useful distinctions the team learned early on is the difference between terror and horror. Terror is anticipatory fear, or expecting something to be awful. Horror is the actual experience being awful. Tough Mudder aims for obstacles that are high terror, low horror. One obstacle, piloted at a race in Pennsylvania in 2011, was a spectacular failure in this regard. The challenge was to eat a habanero pepper. It seemed like it would make a good story, and the team could imagine people including the obstacle in their highlights recap: *I ate a hot pepper!* In reality, people didn't spend much time thinking about it, and they underestimated how much it would hurt. Most participants just picked the habanero up, popped it in their mouth, and kept running. "The terror was very low and the horror was extremely high," Kombol recalls. The lesson was learned, and now the team looks for ways to widen the terror/horror gap in the opposite direction. (They also try out any new obstacle with employees first.) When testing new challenges, the design team has people rate their fear going in and their fear coming out. They're looking for experiences that transform terror into triumph. That's how you end up feeling like a hero.

When Cathy Merrifield stood on the twelve-foot-high platform debating whether to jump, she was facing one of the most important aspects of a Tough Mudder obstacle: the decision point. Kombol's team tries to create what he calls the "Holy shit, I'm about to do this!" moment for every obstacle. They want participants to pause and think about what they're about to do. When Victor Rivera, a personal trainer in Los Angeles, faced the Arctic Enema—a dumpster filled with eight thousand pounds of ice—in his first Tough Mudder, he said to himself, "You know, you can walk around this. They don't force you to do the obstacles." As he considered skipping the ice bath, he realized it was a metaphor. "Life is filled with crossroads, where you decide to continue on the path toward your goals or give up in the face of adversity." He decided he would rather test himself than regret passing it up. "Even though I was an ice cube for the next twenty minutes, I was glad I stepped up to the plate. It's carried over into my weight lifting, academics, and even parenting," he told me. "Whenever I feel that I've reached my limit, I know that there's more in there."

The single obstacle that gives Mudders the most pause is Electroshock Therapy, a twenty-by-forty-foot maze made out of curtains of electrified wires. A 10,000-volt bolt of electricity zaps through the wires thirty times per minute. The obstacle is out in the open, with no walls, so participants can see people running through and getting shocked. Most stand outside for a while, watching, before they enter. "You see last-minute hesitations, absolute fear and dread," Kombol told me. "That hill that you have to get over with yourself is the big one." For most participants, it's this psychological barrier more than any physical one that defines the Tough Mudder experience. And again, that's by design. "It's not 'I went to Tough Mudder and I was on a conveyor belt, and they put me through a series of electrified wires,' which could be one way to do it," Kombol says. "It's 'I went up to this obstacle, I thought about whether I wanted to do it or not.' You get a choice to say I do or I don't."

For years, Electroshock Therapy was the final obstacle on the course, the event designed to leave the lasting impression. It differs from many of the most feared obstacles in that it delivers on the dread. The shocks are real, and Mudders who make it through will tell you, *Yes, it really hurts.* Why make this the last part of the hero's journey? As I thought about the psychology of this obstacle, I became fascinated by its similarities to a specific series of laboratory experiments conducted on rats. In these studies, experimenters deliver electric shocks to rats by attaching an electrode to their tails or through an electrified grid on their cage floor. If you shock rats in an unpredictable and unavoidable manner, you can trigger behaviors that look like depression, anxiety, or post-traumatic stress disorder. The rats become less interested in eating or socializing with other rats. They freeze at any unknown noise or sign of threat. And having learned that there is nothing they can do to prevent the shocks, they stop trying to improve their situation in other stressful contexts—a phenomenon known as *learned helplessness.* Throw the rats in a bucket of water and they won't even try to swim, sinking to the bottom in what psychologists call a *defeat response*.

But sometimes shocking rats doesn't make them helpless; instead, it makes them confident, even courageous. The key to reversing the psychological effect of shocks is to give the rats some element of control. *Any* element of control. For example, in one setup, a rat is placed in a running wheel with an electrode attached to its tail. The experimenter delivers shocks until the rat turns the wheel. The rat can't prevent new shocks, but it can shorten their duration. This rat doesn't become depressed or traumatized; it becomes braver in new environments and more resilient to future stress.

Some researchers believe that what gets learned through controllable shocks is a different relationship to fear. What the rat learns isn't "Shocks are okay." It's not even "Wheels are good." What the rat learns is "I can do something." Fear means *act*, not *freeze*. When Tough Mudders run through Electroshock Therapy, what they learn isn't "I love being shocked" or even "I can survive pain." It's "I am brave." This is something Cathy Merrifield took away from her Tough Mudder experience, after she found the courage to jump off the twelve-foot platform into the water below. "Any kind of physical practice where you push yourself, when you make it past that, you build a confidence in yourself. If you allow it, it lasts, and you can call on that in the next difficult situation in your life. How much can you push yourself? Where's the end? You realize, I don't know that there is."

Many Tough Mudder obstacles require teamwork. To get through the Block Ness Monster, eight people in a pool must coordinate their efforts to rotate, then fling their bodies over, massive blocks in water. In Hold Your Wood, teams carry a giant log over and under a series of obstructions, recalling the cooperative log races performed by indigenous tribes in Brazil. Everest is a curved ramp coated with vegetable oil or dish soap. When you run up the ramp, participants who have already made it to the top reach out to catch you and keep you from slipping back down.

Early Tough Mudder events didn't have a lot of teamwork built in; that element evolved from seeing how participants came together to deal with unexpected challenges. The first time lead obstacle designer Nolan Kombol witnessed spontaneous collaboration was at an event in New Jersey, as participants tried to run up a ten-foot-high mud hill. It had rained that morning, and the mud was as slick as a sheet of ice. No one could make it up the hill. The participants started working together, taking off their shirts and tying them together to create rope ladders. Afterward, everyone was hugging and high-fiving one another. "It was fantastic, better than anything I could have thought of," Kombol remembers. The impromptu teamwork that day led to the creation of Pyramid Scheme, in which people form human ladders to pull other Mudders up and over a slanted wall.

It turns out people like overcoming challenges together, and teamwork obstacles bring out a different side of participants. "When you see a person you don't know who needs your hand, it's pretty serious—'I got you. I want to help you.' On the receiving end, people are grateful. It's meaningful," Kombol told me. "I've spent hours watching people on these obstacles, watching how serious people get in that moment. It's not panic, but it's 'I need to focus,' a human focus. The more I've observed it, the more I watch it, the interaction between strangers—people crave it."

Kombol's description made me think of the stories that get widely shared after a natural disaster—tales of ordinary citizens revealing themselves to be heroes by helping strangers, carrying people to safety, and returning to rescue those left behind. We are inspired by these examples, but many of us also wonder: Would that be me? In that situation, would I turn out to be an unexpected hero? When I mentioned to Kombol how significant it might be to witness your own willingness to grab a stranger's hand and carry them over a wall, he agreed, but then pointed out that it's equally important to the person being helped. We don't just want to know we can be that person. We also want to believe that those people exist.

Once a year in the small village of San Pedro Manrique, Spain, thousands gather at midnight to watch local villagers walk barefoot over coals burning at 1250 degrees Fahrenheit. People thrill to the display of courage. The fire-walkers are celebrated not only for their ability to withstand pain but also for the fact that they carry a loved one on their backs. Once the crossing is complete, the crowd cheers, and family and friends rush to embrace them both. Researchers who studied the San Pedro Manrique ritual have analyzed the emotions expressed by both the fire-walkers and those they carry. As the fire-walkers cross the coals, their faces show determination, even anguish. But the expressions of their loved ones are pure happiness. Part of what draws us to physical challenges like Tough Mudder is the opportunity to see ourselves as the valiant hero. But perhaps, less obvious, is the chance to be rescued. To let ourselves be lifted up and carried by others.

Humans are not the only species to help one another. Bottlenose dolphins will swim underneath a sick dolphin and push its head above water to help it breathe. When a Seychelles warbler becomes entangled in a seed cluster, fellow birds pick the sticky seeds out of its wings until it is able to fly free. An ant attacked by termite soldiers, limbs torn off in the struggle, will be carried back to its nest by other ants in its colony. In the wild, such aid is always preceded by a call for help. Sick dolphins emit two short whistles. Stuck warblers trill an alarm call. Injured ants release distress pheromones. We humans—so used to hiding our weaknesses or minding our own business—sometimes need to practice this call and response: "I'm here, and I need help." "I'm here, let me help you." When such heroic helping occurs in nature, the individual being rescued tends to be one of high value to the group or to the one doing the helping. Whether you are an ant, a bird, or a dolphin, you get saved because you matter. Perhaps this, too, is one of the joys of events like Tough Mudder: the feeling of *I matter*. There's the story we tell on social media, exuberant and boastful—"I ran through electrified wires!" And there's the story we remember later, with gratitude. *When I reached out a hand for help, someone grabbed it.*

• • •

In the early 1800s, philosopher Thomas Brown argued that our muscles constitute an "organ of sense" through which we come to understand ourselves as individuals. Through movement and muscular contraction, we literally sense our "self" as someone who exists in and interacts with the world. Brown was anticipating the scientific discovery, nearly a century later, that every time you move your body, sensory receptors in your muscles, tendons, and joints send information to your brain about what is happening. This is why if you close your eyes and raise one arm, you can feel the shift in position and know where your arm is in space. You don't have to watch what's happening; you can *sense* yourself.

The ability to perceive your body's movements is called *proprioception*, from the Latin roots for "one's own self" and "to grasp." Proprioception, sometimes referred to as the "sixth sense," helps us move through space with ease and skill. But it also plays a surprisingly important role in self-concept—how you think about who you are and how you imagine others see you. The regions of your brain that produce your sense of self-awareness (this is "me") receive signals from your muscles and joints, as well as your heart, lungs, gut, and even the jiggling of crystals in your inner ear that track your relationship to gravity. All of these internal sensations contribute to your broader sense of "me-ness." At some very basic level, you know who you are because your body tells you, *This is your arm reaching, this is your leg kicking, this is your spine rotating, this is your heart beating.* In neurological disorders where proprioceptive feedback is impaired, a person can look at their own arm waving and wonder if it is a stranger's. As one person with impaired proprioception notes, "My limbs just feel lost . . . like someone else's shadow."

The importance of proprioception in constructing your self-image goes far beyond knowing that your arm is *your* arm. When you participate in any physical activity—sports, dance, running, weight lifting—your moment-to-moment sense of self is shaped by the qualities of your movement. When you move with grace, your brain perceives the elongation of your limbs and the fluidity of your steps, and realizes, "I am graceful." When you move with power, your brain encodes the explosive contraction of muscles, senses the speed of the action, and understands, "I am powerful." When you move in a way that requires strength, your brain senses the resistance in your muscles and the force on your tendons, and concludes, "I am strong." These sensations offer convincing data about who you are and what you are capable of. My twin sister once told me that her favorite part of a run is "the part when it's horrible." When I laughed, she explained, "It's a primal feeling. I'm doing this thing that is really tough, and I'm still doing it. *I'm* tough."

Often we are drawn to physical activities that reveal a new side of ourselves. Pamela Jo Johnson never enjoyed exercise until she discovered kettlebells the year she turned fifty, in a class offered in the cafeteria of a local elementary school in Minneapolis. Johnson describes the kettlebell power swing as "the greatest pleasure I have ever known with movement." Johnson likens setting her stance to foreplay. She roots her feet hip-width apart and grips the horn of the forty-four-pound kettlebell in both hands, arms hanging straight down. "The combination of the two-handed grip and the resistance of the weight makes me feel like I am taking on a giant," she told me. She hinges at her hips and leans forward, keeping her chest open and shoulders back. Then she swings the bell backward through her legs and, with a loud exhalation, braces her core, pushes down through her legs, and propels the kettlebell forward and up. "It's such a simple move, but it's a total body movement that packs strength, balance, and grace. I feel powerful and euphoric."

About a month after I chatted with Johnson, she posted a photo on Facebook of a tree toppled by a thunderstorm and blocking two lanes of traffic. Johnson had been in a cab on her way to the airport, and the cars ahead of them were crossing the median and turning back. "My cabdriver and I decided we would work our way to the front and see if we could move it," she wrote. Two other women and four men joined them to help move the tree. When I saw her Facebook post, I immediately pictured Johnson swinging a kettlebell. Every time Johnson swings that bell, sensations of power infiltrate her self-perception. And once you've sensed yourself as powerful, it changes the way you look at an obstacle in your way. Would Johnson have thought of herself as someone who could move a tree without the experience of kettlebell training? I sent her a message asking if she thought there was a connection. "When the tree presented itself, I felt invincible," she wrote back. It was as if her nervous system took stock of the fallen tree, recalled the euphoric feeling of swinging a forty-four-pound bell, and remembered that she is someone who can take on a giant.

If there is a voice in your head saying, "You're too old, too awkward, too big, too broken, too weak," physical sensations from movement can provide a compelling counterargument. Even deeply held beliefs about ourselves can be challenged by direct, physical experiences, as new sensations overtake old memories and stories. Strength trainer Laura Khoudari, who works with people who have a history of psychological trauma, observes, "I have seen women who have felt small for years, not just because of their stature, but because of their circumstances, lift more weight than they had ever considered possible, and then walk out of the gym a bit more empowered. . . . Picking up more than you thought you could, can very literally show you that you can handle more than you think you can."

Katie Norris, a Unitarian Universalist minister and CrossFit coach, found this kind of revelation through a movement called the *partner carry*. It's an exercise in which you run with another person thrown over your shoulder or clinging to your back.

(CrossFit is popular with firefighters, emergency responders, and the military, for whom this is an extremely relevant skill.) When Norris joined her local CrossFit in Cleveland, Ohio, "My assumption was my body just couldn't do it, so I would never try it." Whenever the partner carry showed up in a daily workout, she carried a sandbag instead. It wasn't just the required strength that worried her; it was also the close physical contact with another person. "Part of it was the whole living up to whatever a woman is supposed to look like. I've never been that. I'm shorter, bigger, sweatier. I always felt ashamed of my body."

As Norris continued to train at CrossFit, she got stronger, developed new skills, and practiced going outside her comfort zone. Her husband and son also joined, often training with her at the gym. When her family moved to Richmond, California, they found another CrossFit box. But for seven years, she never attempted the partner carry. In her mind, it was off-limits, beyond the realm of what was possible. Then one summer, when class was held on the beach, the list of that day's exercises included a fifty-meter partner carry. Her husband was there to partner with her, and Norris thought, *It's just sand, so if I drop him, it won't be that bad.* She told herself to listen to what was real in that moment, instead of listening to all the old stories in her head about what was wrong with her body and what she could or couldn't do. As her husband climbed onto her back, she took a deep breath, braced the muscles of her core, and pitched forward. With her husband's arms wrapped around her chest, her arms pulling him close, she carried him across the sandy beach. Her son, who was twelve at the time, took a picture, and in it, Norris looks determined, like the fire-walkers of San Pedro Manrique.

When she reached the fifty-meter mark, she was amazed. "It's weird, because I literally carried someone, but it felt instead like a weight was lifted off," she told me. "All the bad stuff I had assumed would happen, the stuff I thought I couldn't do, that was gone. There was a sense of relief. And I was just proud." Norris has since done the partner carry with strangers, and she describes the experience as both empowering and humbling. "Because I'm a minister, I see things in a spiritual way. Some-body trusts you to carry them, which is an honor. I feel a pro-found sense of responsibility. It makes me a little bit nervous, but it also makes me feel strong."

The transformation Norris felt from this breakthrough is part of what led her to become a CrossFit coach. "For me, minis-try is about helping people find their path in life by being fully who they are. There is a deep process in physical movement that is a finding of one's self—mentally, emotionally, physically, and in relation to the universe." Recently, Norris was coaching a woman in a deadlift, an exercise where you pick up and then lower a weighted barbell. It looks simple, but deadlifts can be intimidating. It's not unusual for people to spend more time psyching themselves up for the movement than it takes to per-form it. In an online forum dedicated to strength training, one weight lifter described how his heart will be perfectly calm as he stands in front of the barbell, but the moment he touches the bar, it races into full fight-or-flight mode. As Norris was coach-ing this woman in the deadlift, she noticed signs of fear on the woman's face and in her posture. Norris had previously ob-served that the woman had a habit of putting her arms around her belly when she felt vulnerable, something you can't do while lifting a barbell. So she talked the woman through the proper method of bracing her core, the same technique Norris had used to steady herself for her first partner carry. Then she encouraged the woman to think about that physical action as a way to support herself. "Think of it as putting your arms around yourself, but with your own muscles." The metaphor of supporting herself worked, and as the woman lifted and lowered the heavy weight, new sensations of inner strength and self-care entered her muscle memory.

I remember having a similar discovery when I was in my twenties, with a yoga backbend known as king pigeon pose. To enter the pose, you stand on your knees, press your palms together at your heart, and lean backward slowly, until just the crown of your head touches the floor behind you. For someone like me, who likes to know what's happening at all times, the blind entry can be terrifying. Without the muscle control to slow your descent, you crash-land on your head. It's the kind of physical risk I would typically avoid, but there was something about the entry to this pose that captivated me. It was like a trust fall, except the person I had to trust was myself. What would catch me was my own strength.

It took me over a year of practice to be able to do the pose. For a long time, I asked a partner to stand in front of me and brace my hips as a kind of safety net. When I finally did the movement on my own, I felt like someone I didn't quite recognize—a person who might head willingly and wholeheartedly into some unknown adventure. That was almost twenty years ago, but I can still remember the feeling of falling backward, opening my heart, and sensing my strength. My yoga practice has changed as my body has, and it's been years since I last tried that backbend. I don't know if I could still do the pose, but the memory, the sensation, and the lesson have never left me.

One of the first things you notice at DPI Adaptive Fitness in Fairfax, Virginia, is the Wall of Greatness. The wall, which stretches across the long side of the 1300-square-foot gym, has become a canvas for motivational phrases like "Believing is achieving," "NOT dropping first," and "3rd and 3, give it to me." Anyone can work out at DPI, but the gym specializes in training people with physical challenges. Many have had a stroke, a spinal cord injury, or a limb amputation. The vibe of the gym is, to put it bluntly, badass. On any given day, you might see a young boy with cerebral palsy batter a boxing bag while two women in wheelchairs wage a battle rope competition and a man with a walker uses a harness to drag a tire across the floor. The sound of Pandora's Pop and Hip Hop Power Workout playlist mixes with the trainers' shouts of "Get it!" and "Keep going!" On a pillar in the middle of the room, someone has chalked the words *I don't sweat—I leak awesome!*

I asked thirty-eight-year-old owner and founder Devon Palermo, who with his buzz cut and athletic build looks like he could be leading boot camp, to tell me about the Wall of Greatness. "When we moved into the space, I wanted a way to highlight people's accomplishments," he said. "When new members join, we let them know, if you're willing to work hard, we'll set something very challenging, something you won't be able to do in one or two sessions. If you destroy that goal, you can put up your name and a motivational quote to inspire others in the gym."

I was curious about the stories behind the quotes. Did Palermo remember what people had done to get their names on the wall? He smiled broadly. "I know everyone's." He pointed at "Keep it lit!"—earned by Miss Ruth, a stroke survivor in her midfifties. When Miss Ruth started working out at DPI after physical therapy, she and her trainer set the goal of strengthening her legs to improve her balance and gait. To get on the Wall of Greatness, she had to complete five hundred reps on a squat machine. "In a row?" I asked. "Yes," Palermo said. "Since then, she's hit a thousand."

Research shows that high-intensity training can significantly improve outcomes following a traumatic injury or stroke, even years after the initial trauma. "You need to be safe, but you need to pushed," Palermo explains. One athlete putting in the work at DPI is thirty-five-year-old Joanna Bonilla. On April 1, 2012, Bonilla woke up in severe back pain. She lives with the autoimmune disease lupus, so joint pain was not unusual. But that day, her back hurt so much she had trouble walking. Bonilla's mother convinced her to go to urgent care, where the physician on duty gave her steroids and sent her to the hospital. When she entered the MRI machine that would reveal a lesion on her spine, she could still feel her legs. By the time the scan was complete, she was paralyzed from the waist down.

Bonilla spent months in and out of hospitals and on bed rest, getting chemotherapy, plasma injections, and blood transfusions. Nothing helped, and the loss of mobility was devastating. "I couldn't do anything," she remembers. "My body had betrayed me. It had let me down right in the peak of my life. My legs gave up on me. That's how I felt." After twelve weeks of rehab and learning to use her wheelchair, her physical therapist introduced her to Palermo. "It was the best thing that ever happened to me," she says. "In physical therapy, progress is 'Oh, she lifted her toe.' At the gym, it's lifting a hundred and thirty pounds. It feels good to see results. I have control of that. He helped me not go to that dark place a lot of people go, depression." Palermo encouraged Bonilla to set big goals, including being able to drive again. To do so, she needed to develop the upper body strength to transfer herself from her wheelchair to her car. "I didn't think it was going to happen," Bonilla recalls. "Devon said, 'We're going to make this happen in three months,' and in three months, I was looking at cars."

Her training regime incorporates boxing, and to secure her spot on the Wall of Greatness, Bonilla landed one hundred punches in thirty seconds while sparring with Palermo. "I never thought I was going to be a girl who could throw good punches. To do one hundred punches in thirty seconds is not something everyone can do," she told me. "While I'm throwing those punches, right in the middle of it, you can either give up, or you can keep going and fight through that pain of your arms burning, your shoulders burning. That feels good." For her quote, Bonilla chose "Don't quit." She used to see those words at her old gym, before she became paralyzed. "Before, I would just see it. Now it makes sense."

Her new goal is to walk in leg braces, an outcome that once seemed even more improbable than being able to drive. I asked Bonilla what it meant to be facing the possibility of walking again after six years. "I never thought I'd get to that point," she said. "I should not be able to lift my legs and walk in braces with the diagnosis I have. They don't understand how I'm doing it, but it's getting done." To prepare, she's working on her core strength, and Palermo has issued a pull-up challenge. As part of the U.S. Marines Corps physical fitness test, female Marines must be able to complete at least ten pull-ups in a row to receive the highest possible score. Men must complete twenty-three.

Bonilla's goal is one hundred. "If I'm going to be walking, I need my abs to be strong, my arms strong," she told me. Sometimes when she's doing pull-ups, Palermo challenges her to hold one, and it reminds her of being on the playground as a kid. "I think about my legs when I'm up there. I pretend to kick my legs because I remember when I was younger that it was something I loved to do. I'm not mad at my body anymore. I say to my legs, 'You're taking a break. That's okay. But we're going to make this happen.'"

In 1825, poet Samuel Taylor Coleridge wrote, "Hope without an object cannot live." Modern psychologists have come to a similar conclusion: Humans crave concrete goals and thrive when pursuing specific aims. C. R. Snyder, who conducted the most rigorous scientific analyses of hope, found that this state of mind—so crucial to our ability to persist in the face of life's obstacles—requires three things. The first is a defined goal, that object on which hope lives. The second is a pathway to reach your goal. There must be steps you can take that lead to progress. The third is trusting that you are capable of pursuing that path. You must believe that you have the inner resources and the necessary support to take each step.

One way to think about DPI Adaptive Fitness is that it is an incubator for hope. At DPI, members set meaningful life intentions, like being able to drive or walk. The trainers then provide the pathway by setting concrete physical objectives, like hitting the number of squats or pull-ups that will develop the necessary strength or stamina. The entire environment, from the background music to the attitude of the trainers, is designed to increase members' confidence that their goals can be met. Trainers make sure members notice the gains they make along the way. "In open gym classes, a participant will see someone walking better or able to do something, and for some reason, they always tell the trainers," Palermo says. "I'll say, 'Go tell them! Tell them what you see!'" The trainers also document moments of triumph so they can be shared and celebrated. When Palermo thought Joanna Bonilla was ready to conquer her boxing challenge, he insisted on taking a video. He wanted to make sure Bonilla would be able to watch it later, show it to others, and see how tough she is. "I'm a person who doesn't want to celebrate and hype it up," Bonilla told me. "He videotaped it so I could understand what an accomplishment it was."

DPI also invites friends and family to work out with members, something that can make a training session both more effective and more meaningful. The mere presence of a loved one can change how you perceive a physical challenge and what you able are able to do. One study found that if you are accompanied by a friend, a hill seems less steep than when you face it alone. In 2007, a medical journal documented the case of a sixty-five-year-old man with Parkinson's disease who was unable to walk more than a few steps without losing his balance. He lived in a region of Northern Israel that was regularly hit with Katyusha and mortar rocket attacks, and when the warning sirens went off, he could not run to safety. During one attack, however, his wife was with him, and she grabbed his arm as he stood from his chair. In that moment, he found that he could not only walk but run. Neurologists concluded that it wasn't the urgency of the situation that unlocked his capacity to move, but the fact that the man could literally follow in his wife's footsteps.

The family-and-friends policy at DPI has another benefit: It adds important witnesses to every triumph. When people who are important to you celebrate your achievement, that accomplishment becomes even more significant. André, who contributed "Believing is achieving" to the Wall of Greatness, came to DPI after a brain injury and stroke left him with a significantly slowed gait. It sometimes took him ten minutes to walk from his nearby parking space to the front door of the gym. Palermo gave André an ambitious challenge, a five-minute single-leg stand on his weaker leg to develop his stamina. When André first tried to balance on his weaker leg, he could barely hold the position. But he built his endurance over time, his wife often by his side encouraging him. When André surpassed the five-minute goal and made it onto the Wall, she was there to see and celebrate it.

The physical challenges members undertake at DPI are objectively impressive, and every victory that has landed someone on the Wall has a *wow* quality. Like the overcoming of a Tough Mudder obstacle, it's a story you can tell, a photo or video you can post on social media, something that earns legitimate bragging rights. One young woman recovering from a brain aneurysm had been working on pulling the equivalent of her own body weight on a sled. Once she reached that goal, her brother, one of her biggest supporters, stood on the weighted sled, and she dragged him across the gym, too. I know because I saw the video on Instagram, where it was racking up views and encouraging comments. When Palermo comes up with challenges for new members, he pays attention to their personalities. He tries to come up with things that are uncommon and that—disability or not—most people cannot do. He looks for the goal that makes someone light up. Something that, when they complete it, will provide undeniable proof of both their progress and their potential.

In *The Anatomy of Hope*, physician Jerome Groopman defines hope as "the elevating feeling we experience when we see—in the mind's eye—a path to a better future." Hope of the kind incubated at DPI can provide a real training edge. In one experiment, psychologists induced hope by asking participants to think of a time in the past they had accomplished an important goal, and how this could help them pursue future goals. Each participant then held one hand in a bath of ice water for as long as they could stand it. The hope induction helped participants stick it out a full minute longer. Think of the difference one minute might make when you are doing pull-ups or balancing on your weaker leg, and every extra second of effort opens the possibility of doing more tomorrow. Further, when people perceive a painful physical exercise as helping them reach their goals, their brains release higher levels of endorphins and endocannabinoids, the chemicals responsible for an exercise high. You can recruit your built-in neurobiological capacity to persist through pain and fatigue if you know what you are reaching for and believe that what you are doing matters.

The importance of hope is why the Wall of Greatness is the first thing new members see when they enter the space and why it's visible from every corner of the gym. It is an ever-present reminder that goals in the gym get met. For those already on the Wall, it's evidence of what they have accomplished. For new arrivals, the Wall invites them to imagine what might be achievable. The first time I spoke with Joanna Bonilla, she told me about a conversation that had taken place at the gym the night before. A new member, a stroke survivor in his fifties, had asked a trainer, "What do I have to do to get on the Wall?" Bonilla says, "He was looking at the Wall, and I could see him literally picking out where he wanted his quote. He was like, 'This is going to happen. My name's going to be on there.'"

ONE OF MY FAVORITE TELEVISION SHOWS is *American Ninja Warrior*, a competition in which contestants from all walks of life run an obstacle course that requires tremendous strength and skill. Something odd happens when I watch the show. My body instinctively tries to lend a hand to the contestants. If they are struggling to maintain their balance or grip, my core braces, as if to help them hold on. If they're preparing to make a big dismount, I'll lean into the side of the sofa, as if throwing my weight to support their landing. When I first caught myself doing this, it struck me as a bit ridiculous, but also delightful. Just watching the athletes and rooting for their success triggered a sympathetic mimicry.

Movement has a potent ability to trigger a sympathetic response in an observer. Your own heart accelerates as you watch a baseball player sprint toward home base. Your stomach lurches when you see a skydiver jump out of a plane. When a runner crosses the finish line and throws his fists in the air, you let out a triumphant cheer. This embodied empathy is surely part of the thrill of watching sports, dance, or stunts. As writer Jonah Lehrer observes, "When I watch Kobe glide to the basket for a dunk, a few deluded cells in my premotor cortex are convinced that I, myself, am touching the rim. And when he hits a three pointer, my mirror neurons light up as if I've just made the crucial shot." I would argue this perception is not so much a delusion as an evolutionary advantage. The human capacity for empathy is rooted in the mirror neuron system and its ability to observe and interpret the physical actions of others. Your body responds sympathetically to another person's movement because humans instinctively try to understand one another.

In addition to the pleasure such empathy can afford, it is also a way to broaden our sense of what is possible for ourselves. As dance critic John Joseph Martin wrote in 1936, "When we see a human body moving, we see movement which is potentially producible by a human body and therefore by our own." When you watch others move, you don't just perceive their action. You *proprioceive* it. You receive it into yourself. This is what empathy does: It creates, in your mind, a felt sense of what you are observing. When you watch an athlete compete, a dancer perform, or a child play, you sense their actions in your own body, even if you aren't always aware that's what's happening. This makes observing movement more than a visual experience; it's also a visceral experience. When you sense, empathically, the movement of others, you also sense that movement as part of your "self." Our bodies learn what is possible by seeing and *sensing* the strength, the speed, the grace, and the courage of others. I think this is one reason I found myself watching so many videos of Tough Mudder events and athletes training at DPI Adaptive Fitness. It was more than research. It was inspiration. Not just in some sentimental or cerebral way, but in a deeply embodied way. Allowing yourself to be moved by the actions of others is a way to catch hope.

At the CrossFit box where Reverend Katie Norris coaches, the gym has a personal record board. Every time someone gets a faster time, lifts a heavier weight, or masters a movement they could not do before, that person gets to write it on the board and ring a bell. When the bell rings, the whole gym stops what they're doing to cheer. "It often happens that a workout is so hard that someone is not sure they can finish it," Norris told me. "We all gather around them and cheer them on, and when they are done, they fall to the ground crying, and we hug them."

I don't think it's a coincidence that so many people are drawn to communities where they can pursue physical challenges along-side others. It is a joy to watch people exert themselves, face their fears, and overcome obstacles. At Norris's gym, members some-times show up just to witness what others are accomplishing. "When someone in the midst of a depressive episode comes in and just sits and watches class because they could barely get themselves out of the door and into the car, that is beautiful." This is also how collective hope works. Sometimes you are the one crushing the goal and ringing the bell. Sometimes you get to be part of the crowd that hugs and cheers the person ringing the bell. And sometimes it's enough to simply immerse yourself in a space where such a joyful noise gets made.

Four months after my first conversation with Joanna Bonilla, I stopped by DPI Adaptive Fitness in Fairfax, Virginia. When we had last spoken, Bonilla was just beginning to imagine the pos-sibility of walking in leg braces. It had seemed an unlikely goal for so long, but her training was making it possible. Even though I knew how hard Bonilla was working, I was not prepared for what I saw when we met up. After completing her regular work-out in her wheelchair, she took out two custom leg braces. One at a time, she strapped the braces around her thighs and shins, inserted her feet into the curved white plastic footholds, and laced up her black sneakers. Then she stood, gripped the handles of a walker, and walked across the gym floor.

When Bonilla agreed to talk to me about her experience training at DPI, she wanted to use a pseudonym. That's not uncommon. Many people are happy to share their stories but don't want a public spotlight. Even her quote on the Wall of Greatness uses a nickname—it's attributed to *T.N.*, or "the nerd," because Bonilla is always pushing for more knowledge, always asking the trainers at DPI to explain why. But after our conversation, Bonilla changed her mind and gave me permission to use her full name. "It's not fair for me to hide myself," she said. "I want people to learn from my experiences and be able to contact me if they need encouragement to do something they are scared of." In her decision to use her real name, she seemed to me to be at the top of some obstacle, reaching out. Wanting to grab a stranger's hand, pull them up, and carry them over.

Chapter 6

EMBRACE LIFE

When I spoke with Susan Heard about running, she was in her home office in Easton, Pennsylvania. The forty-six-year-old mother of two works as a major gift officer for St. Baldrick's, a childhood cancer research foundation. Her office is decorated with shadow boxes that display medals and photos from 5Ks and half marathons she has participated in. Hundreds of colorful paper origami cranes also hang from the walls, strung together in cascading chains. The cranes—meant to be a message of hope—were her son David's project. Before he died from cancer at the age of ten, David had wanted to have mobiles of cranes installed in every children's hospital in the United States.

David was eight when the doctors discovered the neuroblastoma wrapped around his kidney, aorta, and vena cava. On the ultrasound, it looked like the tumor was strangling his heart. A neighbor offered to make special rubber bracelets—similar to the LiveStrong yellow bands so popular at the time—that the community could wear to support David and his family. Heard asked David what he wanted the bracelets to say, and he decided,

"Embrace life." The family did their best to honor these words. There was chemotherapy, surgery, and radiation, but also backyard Nerf battles, family vacations, and dance parties in the kitchen. When David was invited to share his story at a fundraiser, he surprised Heard by announcing to the crowd, "To kick things off, we're going to have my mom shave her head!"— and so she did. It felt empowering. Then the cancer came back, and the medical options ran out. David died on February 10, 2011, and Heard fell into a deep depression.

Almost four years after her son died, she sat on her couch on New Year's Eve, thinking, *I'm not even alive. Why am I here?* "I was in so much pain. I didn't want to be alive," she remembers. As those thoughts echoed in her mind, she asked herself, *Is that really true? Do I really not want to be alive?* Her husband had gotten her a Fitbit for Christmas, so she decided, *Maybe if I start exercising, I'll feel better.* "I kept telling people, 'Embrace life.' I was saying the words, but I was not doing it," she told me. "I was just trying to find a way to get back."

Heard started to walk the family dog more often. She worked her way up to thirty minutes on an elliptical machine. Within a year, she joined a local running group. The leader who set the group's pace slowed the entire pack when Heard first joined, so she wouldn't feel left behind. "I was too new to running to even know," Heard says. "That group got me through it." They run outdoors in all seasons, along a six-mile loop at a local fish hatchery. "There's something about being outside, something peaceful. There's something about being with the weather, the sun, the wind, all of that. It's a different sense of being alive, being connected to your world. I feel I see more, I know more, about my world."

It was during these outdoor runs that Heard started to experience something unexpected. "I'm often looking for David," she told me. "I've had moms who've said, 'I dream about my child.' The only dreams I've ever had about David are horrible, the horrible things that happened." While running, she started to feel his presence. "There are these moments when you get into this state of true relaxation. Your body is working, but your mind lets go. When I run, and I get there in my head, I feel him," she says. "A fox runs in front of me, a cardinal dodges out of a branch, a squirrel acting bizarre—you notice these things out there. My immediate connection is always, 'Hi, David.' That's how I feel. He's showing me that he's here. When it happens, it's tremendous. We're always looking for these opportunities to feel them or to see them. And for me, that's where I've found him. Outside."

Psychologists call physical activity that takes place in a natural environment *green exercise*. Within the first five minutes of any physical activity in nature, people report major shifts in mood and outlook. Importantly, they don't just feel better—they feel different, somehow both distanced from the problems of every-day life and more connected to life itself. Taking a walk out-doors slows people's internal clocks, leading to the perception of time expanding. Simply being in an environment with a va-riety of plant species increases people's ability to gain perspec-tive on their lives. Even just remembering a time spent in the presence of natural beauty makes people more likely to say they feel connected to the world around them, unburdened by every-day concerns, and in the presence of something greater than themselves.

Spending time outdoors can also calm an agitated mind. The

emotions we are most likely to feel in nature—wonder, awe, curiosity, hope—are natural antidotes to worry, distraction, and depression. As one man describes the internal state he felt while canoeing through Canada's wild rivers, "There were no sharp things inside me . . . not a sense that something was wrong, or I needed to work on something, there was just a peace, there was tranquility, there was acceptance, there was harmony." Others report finding in nature "a complete sense of belonging" and a feeling of being held, "similar to when you really genuinely hug a person." The psychological benefits of outdoor activity can be profound. At the Hong-reung Arboretum in Seoul, Korea, middle-aged adults being treated for depression walked among the trees and alpine plants before participating in their weekly cognitive behavioral therapy sessions. At the end of one month, 61 percent of the forest-walkers were in remission, three times the rate of patients whose psychotherapy took place in a hospital. In an Austrian study, adding mountain hiking to standard medical treatment reduced suicidal thinking and hopelessness among individuals who had previously attempted suicide.

Our tendency to spend most of our days indoors is a relatively recent reversal. The human brain evolved over a long period of history when humans spent most of their time outdoors, interacting with the natural world. Because of this, the human mind responds to nature in ways that bring out many of our cognitive strengths. Being active outdoors can help us tap into the human capacity for mindfulness, as well as the transcendence of being connected to something bigger than ourselves. It puts us in touch with the innate joy that biologist E. O. Wilson calls *biophilia*, or love of all that is living. It helps us see our own lives from a broader point of view. Understanding how green exercise achieves these effects can teach us something important about the human mind—both how it can get stuck in a cycle of suffering and how we can find peace.

• • •

One cold February afternoon, writer Maura Kelly left her Brooklyn apartment, not sure where she was going, but knowing she had to get out. Kelly had lived with depression for years, but her despair had been escalating as one thing after another fell apart: a relationship ending, a string of professional disappointments, a sleep disorder that left her exhausted. The day she fled her apartment, Kelly was trying to escape the prison her mind had become and the thoughts that tormented her: *I'm not good enough. I will never be happy. I'll always be alone. All my effort will come to nothing.*

She found herself walking the sloping hills of Fort Greene Park, a thirty-acre urban forest filled with Norway maples, American elms, and Austrian pines. She was the only person braving the bitter cold. Among the trees and fresh air, Kelly felt something shift. As she would later write in an essay, "I felt more free, less trapped in my apartment and in my head. . . . instead of being taunted into one dark corner after another by the voices in my head, I went one way, round and round, and turtled deep in my jacket, felt better able to listen to what was good in myself." Inside her apartment, she had felt completely immersed in her negative thoughts. It was as if her worries and self-judgments filled the space around her and became the very air she was breathing. "Outside," she told me, "I was around more positive thoughts. Like, 'Ah, the big sky, the big trees, the air—this is good. I'm okay. I'm still alive. I'm free.'"

Unlike a runner's high, the mind-altering effects of green exercise kick in almost immediately. These fast-arriving benefits cannot be explained by the slow accrual of feel-good chemicals like endocannabinoids or endorphins. Instead, it's as if being in nature flips a switch in the brain to transport you into a different state of mind. The question is, what switch? If neuroscientists had been able to observe what was happening in Maura Kelly's brain as she walked through Fort Greene Park, they almost certainly would have detected a change in the *default mode network*. This brain network was first identified twenty years ago, when researchers used functional neuroimaging to document the baseline state of an awake human brain. Before then, brain-imaging studies had focused on figuring out which brain structures are active during specific tasks. Neuroscientists would scan people's brains while asking them to solve math problems, memorize word lists, or analyze the emotions expressed in photographs. Eventually some of these researchers thought to ask: What happens in the brain when a person is lying in a brain-imaging machine waiting for instructions? What does the brain do when you're not doing anything and the mind is allowed to wander?

When neuroscientists analyzed the brain's baseline state, the answer surprised them. The resting brain turns out not to be resting at all. Many systems throughout the brain are active, including those linked to memory, language, emotion, mental imagery, and reasoning. Even more stunning was the finding that all human brains, at rest, slip into a similar state. Neuroscientists dubbed this pattern of brain activity the *default*. Left to its own devices, the human mind holds imaginary conversations, replays past experiences, and reflects on the future. It especially likes to think about you, your goals in life, and your relationships with others. This default state is essential for functioning in a social world. The brain's baseline activity is also how we remember who we are. Its inner chatter and imagery provides the awareness that you exist as a specific individual, with preferences, aspirations, and problems, one who continues across time and context. You wouldn't want the alternative—a brain that struggles to create a coherent sense of self or place in the world. That is what happens in late-stage Alzheimer's disease, when pathological tangles ravage the core structures of the default network.

However, the default state also has a downside. For many of us, the mind's default has a negative bias. Its most familiar habits are to ruminate on past hurts, criticize ourselves or others, and rehearse reasons to worry. The default state can also become a mental trap. In theory, when you focus on something—a conversation, a movie, work—the default mode quiets down and allows the brain to enter a state of outwardly directed attention. But people who suffer from depression or anxiety don't make this switch as easily. They show unusually high activity in the default mode network, and they get stuck in the default state, making it difficult to focus on anything or anyone else, or even to fall asleep. For some, the mind can even become addicted to rumination. The brain's reward system—not a core part of the default mode network—can become highly connected to the structures within the default mode network that are associated with memories, worry, and thinking about yourself. Every time you revisit a familiar fear or judgment, the reward system says, "Yes, more of that!" It's as though the brain is convinced that some good might come from the rehashing, worrying, or self-criticism. When this happens, you can find yourself as unable to escape these mental habits as a heroin user trying to suppress their cravings and compulsions.

One of the most effective ways to quiet the default state is meditation. In brain-imaging studies, focused breathing, mindfulness, and repeating a mantra have all been shown to deactivate hubs of the default mode network. In one unusual case study, neuroscientists at the Weizmann Institute of Science in Israel studied the brain activity of a sixty-four-year-old meditation master who had spent more than twenty thousand hours meditating. As he moved through different states of consciousness, from a typical default state to a "selfless" state of pure awareness, his brain scan showed the default mode network disengaging.

Green exercise appears to do something similar to the brain, but without the need for such dedicated mind-training. At least one study has tried to capture this effect with brain-imaging technology. Researchers at Stanford University sent participants out on a ninety-minute walk. Some hiked the Dish, a scenic trail in the foothills near campus, while others walked along one of the busiest streets in Silicon Valley. Before and after the walk, neuroscientists put the participants in an fMRI machine to capture their brains' resting activity. The participants also answered questions about their state of mind, including how much they agreed with statements like "My attention is focused on aspects of myself I wish I'd stop thinking about." After the scenic hike—but not the walk on the busy roadway—participants reported less anxiety and negative self-focused thinking. Their post-walk brain scans revealed less activity in the subgenual cortex, an area linked to self-criticism, sadness, and rumination. Individuals who suffer from depression show more activity in this part of the brain during "rest" than people who are not depressed. A walk in nature selectively silenced this part of the default state's stream of consciousness.

Notably, the very same neurological change has also been detected in two of the most promising experimental treatments for depression: transcranial magnetic stimulation, which delivers an electric current to the brain through a magnetic coil on the scalp, and ketamine, an anesthetic used on the battlefield during the Vietnam War and popularized as a recreational drug during 1990s rave culture. Magnetically stimulating the prefrontal cortex reduces the active connections between the subgenual cortex and other brain regions in the default mode network. This change is linked to reduced symptoms of depression among patients who had not responded to any previous antidepressant medications. Intravenous infusions of the drug ketamine disrupts the brain's resting state in precisely the same way. This reorganization of the default mode network, which persists twenty-four hours after being given a dose of ketamine, overlaps with the peak antidepressant effect of the drug.

There's no evidence that these three "therapies"—transcranial magnetic stimulation, ketamine, or exercising outdoors—are interchangeable, and no responsible scientist or health-care provider would encourage someone who is clinically depressed to forgo medical treatment in favor of a hike. Still, it is fascinating that the short-term neurological effect of a walk in a park— something accessible to many people—so closely resembles the mechanism of two cutting-edge treatments for depression. This may explain why the psychological benefits of being in nature are most pronounced among those who struggle with depression. It is also a reminder that making time for physical activity is not self-indulgent. For many, it is an act of self-care, even self-preservation. In his memoir *Dip*, photographer Andrew Fusek Peters—whose father died by suicide—explains how swimming in the rivers, lakes, and waterfalls of Shropshire and Wales interrupted the usual "thought-torture" that defined his own severe depression: "Diving into wild water is the great bringer-back of reality. A perfect present tense, a right-here, right-now moment.

The senses are so filled by the trees, the light, the sound of birds, of shivering leaves, the fierce, squeezing clinch of water—there's no space for thought shadows." Psychotherapy helps him challenge his most self-destructive thoughts, but "it takes an awful lot of cognitive behavior therapy to change the tape." Swimming outdoors turns the tape off.

Peters's description of what he experiences in the water captures something important about how nature affects the mind. When you are absorbed in your natural surroundings, the brain shifts into a state called *soft fascination*. It is a state of heightened present-moment awareness. Brain systems linked to language and memory become less active, while regions that process sensory information become more engaged. The senses are heightened and inner chatter quiets. This shift can be a tremendous relief for people who struggle with anxiety, depression, and rumination, for whom the default mode is relentlessly verbal, generating words and phrases that echo in their minds. By flooding the senses with pleasant stimulation, nature draws your attention outward and interrupts the linguistic assault. There is room for curiosity about and appreciation for the world around you.

Mindfulness practices teach people how to access this state of heightened sensory awareness intentionally. Brain-imaging studies reveal that after people receive mindfulness training, their resting state shifts away from rumination and toward present-moment attention, even while lying in an fMRI machine. Among highly experienced meditators, mindfulness may even replace the usual default mode to become a new baseline state of mind. Meditation teachers like to say that this present-moment focus, including the happiness that comes from it, is the natural state of the mind. To those who live with anxiety or depression, such a claim can seem preposterous. And yet as I learned more about how nature affects the brain, I began to wonder if the human mind has two distinct default modes. There is, of course, the default mode neuroscientists observe when participants are trapped inside a functional imaging machine, a state defined by mind-wandering, self-reflection, and rumination. Might there also be a very different default mode that reveals itself when we are in nature?

Alexandra Rosati, a psychologist who studies the evolutionary origins of the human mind, points out that two pressures shaped the development of the human brain. The first was our need to cooperate in small groups. This pressure gave rise to social cognition, our ability to think about other people. This includes our tendency to define ourselves in relationship to other people and to reflect on our position within our tribe. The second pressure on human evolution was our need to cooperate with the natural environment to find food. According to Rosati, this need gave rise to mental skills she labels *foraging cognition*. Just as natural selection favored anatomical changes—like longer legs and powerful gluteal muscles—that helped humans hunt and gather, it also reinforced mental abilities that helped our ancestors find what they needed. Humans developed a fine-tuned spatial awareness, a mindset open to discovering the possibilities around us, and the patience to continue searching.

As I read Rosati's work, I started to think about how the typical default state is essentially a way to practice the social cognition skills humans developed to thrive in groups. In contrast, the alternate default state of mindfulness—one of open awareness to the environment, with a sense of curiosity and hope—maps onto the "mind" Rosati describes as foraging cognition. Neuroscientists argue that the typical default state exists because humans need to rehearse our social selves to survive as a social species. If this is the case, why wouldn't we also have a default state of mind that reflects our need to engage with nature? For our early ancestors, the ability to explore and find resources in the natural world was as key to their survival as the willingness to share. Surely the human brain evolved to reflect this need as much as it has been shaped by our dependence on one another.

Perhaps the context we find ourselves in determines which default state the mind reverts to. Humans who find themselves disengaged from natural environments may come to know primarily the self-focused default state. Spending time not just indoors, but also on social media, pushes us toward social cognition and, often, rumination. Without regular time spent outdoors, we can lose touch with the default state of open awareness. By reconnecting with nature, we refamiliarize ourselves with this other aspect of what it means to be human. This is a big part of what draws people to green exercise. Outdoors, it is possible to rediscover a self that is not solely defined by your roles and relationships with others, or by your past. You are free to be a self that is in motion, attuned to the present moment, and open to what the world has to offer.

• • •

The psychological effects of physical activity are often compared to mind-altering substances. The runner's high mimics a mild cannabis buzz. Synchronized dancing produces a glow not unlike ecstasy. Moving to music provides an adrenaline rush similar to stimulants. I've even heard a good yoga stretch described as turning one's blood into wine. These comparisons, while imperfect, provide a useful framework for understanding both the appeal and benefits of different kinds of movement. When I began to consider whether such a parallel exists for green exercise, my first thought was that it would have to be some kind of pharmaceutical aimed at anxiety or depression. But if you focus on what is unique about green exercise, the class of drugs it most closely resembles is the entheogen, a category that includes psilocybin, ayahuasca, and LSD. Entheogens are plant-derived substances described by advocates as consciousness expanding, and are ingested to induce a religious or spiritual experience. Like green exercise, these drugs alter consciousness by temporarily reorganizing the default state. During an LSD trip, changes in default network connectivity correlate with the user's feelings of oneness with the universe.

Many people report life-changing insights and moments of self-transcendence while under the influence of these drugs, an outcome that is also surprisingly common for spending time in nature. Eighteen percent of the people in the United States say they have had an intense spiritual experience while in nature, and almost half of all mystical experiences take place in a natural setting. The most common of these experiences is the *unity sensation*, a feeling of union with something bigger than oneself, accompanied by a wave of love and sense of deep harmony. In *Finding Ultra*, Rich Roll recalls such an experience as he ran through the hills of California's Topanga State Park. "I didn't just feel amazing. I felt free. . . . For the first time in my life, I felt that sense of 'oneness' I'd only previously read about in spiritual texts." The unity sensation is often felt as a union with nature itself. One woman, age fifty, experienced just such a diffusion of self while hiking the Grand Canyon in Arizona. "I felt a complete merging with the surrounding environment. Instead of sitting back and observing it . . . it's like I was moving into it in some way, or rather it was moving into me . . . I suppose what I experienced was transcendence, losing myself into my surroundings. It was expansive and at first I was afraid and then deeply comforted and filled with a sense of complete peace."

Researcher Terry Louise Terhaar has conducted in-depth interviews with close to one hundred people about their spiritual experiences in nature. (She notes that while her interviewees declare that what they experienced was indescribable in words, "their command of descriptive adjectives and adverbs often rivals that of the world's great poets"—something author Michael Pollan also noticed about people's attempts to describe their spiritual experiences while under the influence of entheogens.) Terhaar believes that these elevated states of mind confer a survival advantage outdoors. In such a state, she argues, we are more likely to overcome physical pain, fear, or despair. Faced with threats in the natural world, we will find ourselves able to perform heroic feats. The examples Terhaar cites include moving heavy rocks, lifting fallen trees, and escaping unsafe conditions, even if injured. These are all acts that would help us survive the wilderness. According to this logic, modern humans have inherited the ability to be deeply moved while in nature because transcendent states helped our ancestors carry on. Yet it's not hard to imagine that uplifting experiences in nature can be a resource in modern times as well.

Natural environments have the ability to instill feelings of what researchers call *prospect*—an elevated perspective and hopefulness, often triggered by natural beauty or awe-inspiring views—and *refuge*, the sense of being sheltered or protected. Analyses of journal entries written by people during park visits show that the most commonly used words include *love, life, time, world*, and *God*. Reflecting on the psychological benefits of spending time outdoors, psychologists Holli-Anne Passmore and Andrew Howell write: "Connecting with nature embeds us more deeply into the existence of life beyond the course of our single lifetime." This broader point of view can inspire optimism. In one study, walking in a nature reserve for fifteen minutes helped people feel better equipped to handle the challenges in their lives. The more the walk inspired sentiments such as "I can imagine myself as part of the larger cyclical process of living" and "I feel embedded within the broader natural world, like a tree in a forest," the more confident people became that they could resolve their problems.

Several years ago, my husband and I were caring for a terminally ill cat we had rescued twelve years earlier. He had kidney disease, and the medical treatments—daily IV drips, a drug to stimulate his appetite, emergency trips to the vet to remove fluid from his lungs—were distressing and confusing. He would eat only when I fed him by finger, and a successful mealtime might be less than one spoonful over the course of half an hour. A formerly talkative companion, he had stopped meowing altogether. We sometimes found him in the bedroom closet, staring blankly. And yet he still greeted me every morning, sitting on my chest until I woke. He continued to seek our affection and purred when we petted him. Several times a day, he stood by the door to our deck to let me know that he wanted to sunbathe. But he also struggled to sleep, and his breathing was labored. We didn't know if through heroic medical actions, we were extending a life he wanted or just prolonging his misery. The responsibility of having to make this decision for our cat, when he couldn't tell us what he wanted, was overwhelming. We worried both about prematurely ending the life we had vowed to protect and about waiting too long to end his suffering.

My husband and I lived in New York City at the time, and one day, when we were both feeling especially demoralized by the situation, we took a walk in Riverside Park. We passed the fenced play area where off-leash dogs romped and continued through the tunnel that leads to the Hudson River. We walked along the riverfront, taking in the fresh air, blue sky, and lapping of the water. We sat down in a part of the park shaded by trees. It was early autumn, and the leaves had started to change color and drop from the branches. We watched squirrels and sparrows looking for food on the ground. I remember feeling for the first time a sense of perspective on what we were going through. It sounds clichéd, but I recognized that our drama was just one more iteration of a cycle of life that had been playing out for eternity. I realized, with relief, how little control we actually had. I also sensed that our stubborn, steadfast refusal to stop taking care of our cat was a natural instinct to protect, a final burst of fierce, determined love. Our torment was itself part of the caregiving cycle that keeps us alive until it cannot. We returned home that day with a sense that we could handle both the decisions that lay ahead of us and the loss that would soon follow.

• • •

In 2013, the city of Melbourne, Australia, gave the 70,000 trees under its care identification numbers and email addresses. City officials thought they were creating a system for citizens to alert them to maintenance needs, like you might report a pothole, graffiti, or a broken streetlight. They expected residents to inform them of fallen branches or fungal damage. Instead, they were inundated with messages to the trees. The golden elms and weeping myrtles of Melbourne have received thousands of emails expressing affection, kind wishes, and concern for their well-being. When given the chance to communicate with trees, people around the world composed love letters.

The human longing to connect with nature is called *biophilia*, which literally means love of life. According to biologist E. O. Wilson, biophilia is a hardwired instinct that is key to human happiness. The human brain evolved in an environment that was defined by constant contact with and reliance on the natural world. The emotions that modern humans tend to feel in nature—awe, contentment, curiosity, wanderlust—contributed to early humans' ability to thrive as a species that had to find its place in a complex and constantly changing landscape. These emotional responses to nature are still deeply ingrained in us, and the more frequently we experience them, the more fulfilled we are. Across the planet, individuals who feel a stronger connection to nature report greater life satisfaction, vitality, purpose, and happiness. People who make more frequent visits to natural spaces are also more likely to feel that their lives are worthwhile. This effect is even stronger than the benefits of being in good health, and equal to being happily married or living with a partner. One study tracked the daily movements and mood of over 20,000 adults, using the GPS on their smartphones. After collecting over a million data points, the researchers concluded that people are happier in natural environments. And yet typical Americans spend 93 percent of their time indoors, creating what some call a nature deficit.

The need to connect with nature is most evident when humans leave familiar landscapes. Crew members living on the International Space Station, which orbits our planet at 17,000 miles per hour 248 miles above Earth, experience an extreme nature deficit. On board the space station, everything humans take for granted about the natural world is different. The astronauts float weightless, the speed of their vessel untethering them from gravity, our most basic connection to Earth. They go to sleep and wake on a schedule no longer linked to sunrise and sunset. For one week during the space station's orbit, if you turn your head to the right, it is day; look left, and you will see night. The light is unnatural and the air artificial. Astronauts catch a whiff of fresh "space" only when operating the air lock for crewmates returning from spacewalks. They describe the smell of space, which lingers on spacesuits, as metallic, sweet, and reminiscent of welding fumes.

So far from the rhythms, smells, and sounds of their home planet, the crew craves signs of natural life. Many listen to recordings of wind, rain, birds, and even insects. On one expedition, American astronaut and flight engineer Don Pettit decided to try growing a personal garden on the space station. He brought on board packets of seeds from his local corner store in Houston. To make a planter, he stitched together a pair of soiled underwear and sturdy Russian toilet paper, and sewed in a drinking straw connected to a water drip. Pettit wasn't sure the seeds would sprout. After all, there was no sun to stretch toward, no gravity for the first roots to push against. But as he continued his experiments, Pettit's garden began to grow. One of the first seedlings to survive was a zucchini plant, and caring for it—brushing its leaves with a toothbrush, feeding it compost tea brewed from vegetable scraps and orange peels—became the bright spot in Pettit's daily routine. He even took the plant with him when he worked out on the space station's weight-lifting equipment, a makeshift version of green exercise.

The plant became a delight for the entire crew. One fellow astronaut offered to vacuum the station's HEPA filters for Pettit if he could have five minutes with his nose close to the zucchini. The crew became so attached to the plant, they honored it with a call sign—the nickname that fighter pilots are given by their squadron. Space Zucchini, as Pettit had taken to calling it, became Rose, a testimony to how beautiful a vegetable sprout appears in such a sterile environment. NASA's Behavioral Health and Performance team now recommends gardening as a way to protect crew members' psychological health on long missions. As Pettit wrote on NASA's *Space Chronicles* blog, "When you live inside of a metal can filled with machines and electronics, a small splash of growing green is a pleasant reminder from where we came; we all have our roots."

In his 1953 book *Man's Search for Himself*, psychologist Rollo May wrote: "When we relate to nature we are but putting our roots back into their native soil." Although May meant this figuratively, there is evidence that humans need contact with the earth, with dirt itself, to thrive. The bacteria found in ordinary soil can reduce inflammation in the brain, making dirt an antidepressant. When soil gets under your nails in a garden or you breathe deeply in a place where earth is being turned, you expose yourself to these helpful bacteria. The biologists who discovered the benefits of contact with soil named their insight the *old friends hypothesis*. According to this theory, we evolved alongside these microorganisms, and they are vital companions to the human immune system and brain. Just as flowers and bees coevolved and rely on each other, we humans need these bacteria to flourish.

In scientific papers published in microbiology and medical journals, the lack of exposure to dirt in modern society is described as "the loss of old friends"—a loss that is linked in humans to an increased risk of mental suffering, including depression. When you, as psychologist Rollo May describes it, put your roots back into their native soil, it is a cheering reunion. Every time you place your hands in a garden plot, kick up dirt on a running trail, or simply take a deep breath in nature, you harness a biological codependence that has helped humans survive since the earliest days that we lived in groups and learned to depend on one another.

...

When thirty-one-year-old Pete Hutchings first started volunteering at a park in North London six years ago, it was neglected and overgrown. Volunteers would arrive to find drug paraphernalia and empty laptop cases, backpacks, and purses abandoned after robberies. Week after week, they cleared the debris, rooted out invasive species, and tended to the trees. They created pathways for visitors to explore their park and built bug hotels where aphids and butterflies could hibernate. School groups now visit the park every day to learn more about nature. "It's amazing to think how these spaces can transform in a short amount of time," Hutchings says.

Hutchings now manages the park for Green Gym, an initiative in the UK that engages volunteers in conservation-based green exercise. Tasks can include gardening, sowing a meadow, or diggings steps into a clay bank. ("Try digging for twenty minutes, and you'll appreciate the workout this gives," says managing director Craig Lister.) There are local Green Gym teams across England, Scotland, and Ireland, and in the last year alone, volunteers planted over a quarter of a million trees. Each season provides its own satisfying labor. In the summer, volunteers focus on construction, building raised beds for gardening and bird boxes for the coming year. In fall, as nature starts to hibernate, volunteers plant bulbs and make the spaces more accessible to visitors, repairing stairs and building handrails. In winter, they plant young trees that look like dead sticks. Volunteers often ask, "Are you sure these are going to grow?" But then spring arrives, and with it, green buds. Flowers emerge from the bulbs buried in the fall. "It smells new and fresh. Insects are buzzing, and there's the sweet scent of pollen and flowers," Hutchings told me. "It's kind of like the scent of hope after a long dark cold wet winter." Seeing the work come alive months or even years later is one of the most satisfying parts of volunteering with Green Gym. It is the joy of reaping what you sow.

It's not uncommon for volunteers to sign up at a difficult time in their lives. They might be unemployed, be on disability, or have mental health challenges. Green Gym makes it easy to join in. As one volunteer says, "You can just be yourself and are completely accepted." New volunteers get Green Gym T-shirts, a tangible sign that they belong. "We're all pretty scruffy when we're out in the fields. It's okay if you can't afford the latest Nikes," Lister said. "If you show up, you will be welcomed. If you're having a bad day, that's fine, even if you don't want to do much. You can make the tea." The labor of joint tasks allows for a natural companionship, conversations alternating with a comfortable silence that is punctuated by the sounds of wildlife and tools striking earth. The quality of conversation also changes. Being outdoors invites reflection and self-disclosure. In one study, women with breast cancer reported experiencing a "shoulder-to-shoulder support" during green exercise that made talking about difficult topics easier. "What you're saying is almost going into the air, rather than specifically at somebody," one woman observed. "I think that's quite good because you can say things that you might not want to say if you were looking at somebody."

A couple of years ago, Green Gym volunteers put down a piece of lining and some rainwater in a park not far from the central Green Gym office in London. "If you have a small body of water, the wildlife will find it," Hutchings explained. Within a few months, a couple of frogs appeared. Two years later, it is a fully populated pond, with amphibians, dragonflies, tadpoles, and aquatic plants that somehow had all found their way, and, together, turned a puddle of rainwater into a thriving ecosystem. As Hutchings described this to me, I realized that human communities are like this, too. Given a bit of structure—a reason to show up, a place to care for, and time to connect—we build ecosystems of mutual support. The communities that form around movement practices, such as CrossFit, running, group exercise, and recreational sports, are perfect examples of this. And yet collectively cared-for green spaces are especially effective at giving rise to supportive networks. A 2017 analysis of urban community gardens in cities as far-flung as Zagreb, Croatia, Flint, Michigan, and Melbourne, Australia, found that green spaces build social capital. They increase both bonding capital—a sense of belonging, trust, and friendship—and bridging capital, the broad social network you can draw on when you need help. As one member of the North Central Community Gardens in Regina, Canada, explained, maintaining a garden plot opened the doors to becoming much more involved with the neighborhood. "Whereas before it was just my home . . . now this is my community."

The social capital built through gardening can become a shared resource during times of crisis. When Hurricane Sandy struck the Northeastern U.S. in 2012, many parts of New York City were flooded and lost power, including Rockaway Beach, Queens. The Beach 91st Street Community Garden became a central site for distributing food and clothing and sharing news. They kept a fire going so people could stay warm and cook. As one gardener, who described the community garden as "a blanket of support between neighbors," said, "Look at the fifty people eating homemade chili over an open fire two days after one of the most devastating hurricanes in the East Coast. Standing around joking, having hot chocolate . . . when the National Guard can't even get through yet. . . . That is the best defense we have against fear."

E. O. Wilson, the biologist who argued that humans have a hardwired need to connect with nature, also observed, "People must belong to a tribe. They yearn to have a purpose larger than themselves." Green Gym's unofficial tag line is "physical activity with a purpose," and this is how managing director Craig Lister typically pitches the program. "Rather than go to the gym to lift things that don't need to be lifted, give us three hours of the week. At the end of each session, you can stand back, and as a group, you've achieved things." A 2016 National Evaluation of Green Gym found that regular volunteers reported an increase in optimism and feeling useful. They also felt more connected to others and better able to handle the problems in their lives. Spending time in nature and getting more exercise contribute to these benefits, but Lister believes it's the satisfaction of being able to step back and see trees where there weren't any before that does the most good. "We are pack animals who became the world's dominant species, despite all of our frailties, through collaborative effort," he says. "We like to achieve things, particularly as a group, and we love to be valued by the group. We especially love to deliver things as a group when our community values what we have done."

In 2017, researchers at the University of Westminster examined how volunteering for Green Gym affects a physiological index of purpose in life, the *cortisol awakening response*. Although cortisol is best known as a stress hormone, it's also what gets you out of bed in the morning. The cortisol awakening response—measured by the amount of cortisol in your saliva first thing in the morning—helps your body mobilize energy. A sunrise jolt of cortisol brings you out of hibernation and tells you to rejoin the world. People who are depressed or who feel hopeless about the future commonly have a low cortisol awakening response, as if their bodies don't see the point in getting up. Green Gym changes this. After eight weeks of volunteering, Green Gym participants showed a 20 percent increase in their cortisol awakening response, along with a reduction in anxiety and depression. It's as if the experience of tending the green spaces pushed them back out into life.

As the seasons pass, friendships grow, and Green Gym volunteers begin to witness the fruits of their collective labor. The knowledge that they are investing in the future of their communities is part of the appeal of Green Gym. One volunteer, a retired woman well into her seventies, was planting trees with Hutchings. When Hutchings remarked how nice it would be when the trees were grown, she said, "I'm not going to see that. I probably won't be here. But I'm going to take pride in the fact that it will be here for my children and my grandchildren." The volunteers know that what they do matters; by creating and caring for green spaces, they are contributing to the well-being of their communities. In cities as diverse as Delhi, London, and Milwaukee, living in a neighborhood with more green spaces—

including parks and community gardens—is linked to greater life satisfaction and less psychological distress. When the Pennsylvania Horticultural Society turned over two hundred vacant lots in Philadelphia into green spaces by clearing debris and planting grass and trees, the incidence of depression among those who lived nearby dropped by 42 percent.

After a Green Gym project has been going for two years, the organization identifies volunteers who have contributed to their local groups and trains them to become paid leaders. "Green Gym is about moving people to a different place forever," Lister told me. "We changed their lives, and now they help change other people's lives." Eighty percent of current Green Gym employees started as volunteers, including the organization's chief executive, who first volunteered twenty years ago. Pete Hutchings, who started working in a restaurant kitchen when he was thirteen, had no conservation skills or formal education in management when he first volunteered at that neglected North London park six years ago. Now he manages Green Gym projects as a full-time team leader. "I've had many people say the project saved their lives. For people who are struggling, having Green Gym can really pull you through," he told me. "The benefit to people is not why I started, but it's the biggest enjoyment I get out of my job." Even as Hutchings tells me this, it's clear that this part of his job still surprises him, that he is still catching up to his own transformation. "I don't think of myself as a particularly caring person," he said. "I just wanted to be a gardener."

AS THOMAS O. PERRY EXPLAINS in "Tree Roots: Facts and Fallacies," plant roots can grow anywhere. "Root growth is essentially opportunistic in its timing and its orientation. It takes place whenever and wherever the environment provides the water, oxygen, minerals, support, and warmth necessary for growth." Humans have this instinct, too. What E. O. Wilson calls biophilia is not just a love of nature or the tendency to be charmed by birdsong. It is also the will to live, the impulse to grow, and the determination to thrive in whatever circumstances you find yourself in.

Susan Heard, whose son David died from a neuroblastoma at the age of ten, started running outdoors as a way to crawl out of her depression. It has helped her move forward, even as she continues to live with the grief of losing a child. She is embracing life again, just as David wanted. That includes running with her daughter, Daisy, who is now fifteen. "One of the things that I felt the guiltiest about is, I was with David most of the time. She had to grow up a lot, and I wasn't there," Heard told me. "There's a lot of regret, but you have to forgive yourself." One day Daisy surprised her by saying, "I want to try running with you." Heard found a local program called First Strides that coaches women to run a 5K. They completed the ten-week program of outdoor runs together last spring. During one group training session, Heard was at the front of the pack, and she overheard her daughter say with pride to one of the other runners, "That's my mom." Heard's voice came alive as she shared this memory. "Having her with me has been one of the most joyful things."

Chapter 7

HOW WE ENDURE

Shawn Bearden, then forty-two, was running a 50K ultramarathon on Antelope Island near Salt Lake City, Utah. It was his third ultramarathon. The race course promised sightings of wild antelope, deer, coyotes, porcupines, and bighorn sheep. One year a pair of bison blocked the trail a quarter mile from the finish line. ("Go around the animals if you can, or just wait them out," the website advises. "No, you don't get time compensation for buffalo delays.") Unlike some long races that take you through secluded and changing landscapes, the entire Antelope Island course is exposed. The sun beats down with no shade cover. For the second half of the run, you can see the finish line far off in the distance. As Bearden describes it, "It's like that Monty Python movie, where you keep going and going and it's never any closer."

Several hours into the race, he hit a wall of exhaustion worse than anything he had ever experienced. He slowed to a walk. "Every part of me screamed to stop," he remembers. "You feel like you can't move, it's not possible to continue to move, yet somehow you still can. Your muscles feel extremely heavy, like gravity is fifty times stronger than it usually is. That contrast between doing something you know is so simple, just taking another step, and getting all this feedback that this is the hardest thing in the world, leaves your head in a complete state of exhaustion. A helpless exhaustion." Bearden made a deal with himself. He would try to jog for ten minutes. By the time he thought ten minutes had passed, he didn't know if he could keep going, so he said to himself, *If I've made it to seven minutes, I'll force it.* He looked at his watch. It had been one minute. Bearden stopped jogging and started walking again. "Honestly, I was just confused," he recalls.

Runners he had passed on the course were now passing him. Seeing him struggle, they said things like, "Good job, you're going to make it." That helped Bearden keep walking. About half an hour later, without thinking about it, he started to jog again. He had gone a couple of yards before he even realized he was running. The enormous effort it had taken to walk just one step evaporated, and he felt like a ball rolling down a hill. It didn't even feel like he was trying to run; he was just doing it. The momentum carried him all the way to the finish line. "That's when I realized, no matter how bad it gets, I will come through again. I will come back."

Ultra-endurance events are commonly defined as those lasting at least six hours, although many are significantly longer. The Spartathalon in Greece requires athletes to run the equivalent of six marathons in thirty-six hours. The multiday four-thousand-mile Terra Australis Bike Epic takes cyclists down the entire eastern coast of the continent. Competitors in the Iditarod Trail Invitational, an ultramarathon that lasts up to thirty days, must walk, bike, or ski their way through blizzards and gale-force winds from Anchorage to Nome. In recent decades, worldwide participation in such events has exploded. In North America alone, the annual number of individuals who completed an ultramarathon jumped from 650 in 1980 to over 79,000 in 2017.

The oldest official ultramarathon, the 90K Comrades Marathon in South Africa, was founded in 1921 by World War I veteran Vic Clapham to commemorate the hardships of war and the camaraderie of his fellow soldiers. One of the central questions of life is how humans endure the seemingly unendurable, something that, after the brutal Great War, was on Clapham's mind when he founded the Comrades Marathon. According to the event's official history, the annual race "reminds us that through adversity there is hope. Year after year the goodness in humanity comes to the fore."

Today, the ultra-endurance world—in which competitors push their bodies to the limits of what human physiology can withstand—continues to provide a window into both how and why we go on. In *The Lure of Long Distances*, Robin Harvie notes that the word *athlete* derives from a Greek word for "I struggle, I suffer." Ultra-endurance athletes have a relationship to suffering that separates them from most recreational exercisers and that often resembles the wisdom of spiritual traditions. For many, the motivation is not just to complete fantastic feats, but to explore what it means, as one athlete I spoke with puts it, to "suffer well." Their experiences paint a portrait of how humans maintain hope and momentum in the darkest moments. We endure by taking it one step at a time, by making space for suffering and joy to coexist, and with the help of others.

I first reached out to Shawn Bearden, a professor of exercise physiology at Idaho State University, because he produces a popular podcast on the science of ultrarunning. (Ultrarunning is defined as any distance longer than a marathon, but there seems to be no upper limit to what people will try.) Bearden acknowledges that his reasons for getting into the sport might not have been entirely healthy. He has a competitive streak that can be destructive, and there's often a voice in his head arguing that he's not doing enough, something he attributes in part to growing up with a father who was an alcoholic. "I begged him to stop drinking," he told me. "I felt he was choosing that over me." The only thing that got his father's attention was Bearden's success in soccer. So he threw himself into being the best athlete he could be, convinced that if he became good enough, his father would choose him over alcohol. Trying to be the best became his default orientation. "I spent my life trying to be number one at whatever I seemed to have any aptitude at."

Entering midlife, Bearden found himself physically out of shape and judging himself for not staying fit. "I started looking around, thinking, *What can I do?* It's got to be something that other people are going to ooh and aah over." He saw an announcement about an upcoming trail race near where he lived in Pocatello, Idaho. The race had 35K, 60K, and 100K options. He thought, *I've read and heard that only really tough people can survive this.* "So of course I sign up for the 100K, and I had never even run trails before."

He threw himself into training for the event, and when he crossed the finish line, his wife asked, "How do you feel?" "My first word was *happy*," Bearden told me. "It was more like *re-deemed*." He signed up for another race and soon realized how much he enjoyed it—not just the events themselves, but especially the commitment to training that they require. "Twice this week I burst into tears while running," he wrote me in an email. "It's an overwhelming sense of joy that fills me and manifests as happy tears." Later he said, "I've thought a lot about whether I've tried to be the best athlete I can be for reasons that are ultimately negative, or whether I'm doing it for me, because I love it. I'm not one hundred percent sure. But it's in those moments where I break down and feel so happy while I'm running that I realize for sure there is some aspect of this that is for me, that is a healthy and good thing."

Bearden now dedicates much of his free time to helping others prepare for ultramarathons, coaching runners and producing his podcast. "People say a lot of what you learn from ultrarunning can be translated to everyday life, and I've struggled with that," he told me. "Ultrarunning can take you to a place where you strip away everything, and there is nothing left but the essence of you and one thing to do. Keep moving. I'm not sure it has always applied so much to my everyday life. In everyday life, I don't get to a place where the next second is everything I can possibly do," he said. "Except depression. I apply it to my depression."

Bearden has struggled with depression as far back as he can remember. He was only seven years old the first time he thought seriously about killing himself. "I had a plan for it," he explained, then stopped himself from sharing the details. "Well, anyway, it was never going to work." The depression got worse in his teens, and the suicidal thinking stalked him into adulthood. As is the case for many people who struggle with recurrent mental health challenges, the depression—which Bearden describes as "everything feels meaningless, life is pointless, nothing matters"—comes and goes at different periods of his life. He recognizes that he may never be fully free of it. "Depression is a condition that's going to be with me. Coming to accept that is a big step for me," he says. "It's part of who I am, but it doesn't define me."

He describes the onset of an episode as "going dark," explaining, "When it comes, it feels like if you are outside on a nice day and suddenly giant black thunderclouds roll over. You become terrified that the universe has just sat on you, is descending hatred on you. The emptiness is coming in. In those dark moments when the clouds roll in, that funnels quickly into planning suicide." In the past, Bearden would try to outthink the darkness and convince himself that life was worth living. But the more he tried to argue with the worst thoughts, the more logical they seemed. Running, especially outdoors, gives him a way to get out of his head. He calls it "clearing the clouds."

In addition to the mood-stabilizing benefits of training, persisting through an ultra-endurance event holds particular meaning for surviving depression. The perception of time dragging out when you are near physical exhaustion is not unlike what unfolds during depression or grief, when the pain is so bad and the path forward so unclear that you can hardly believe how many moments of suffering a minute can hold. When researchers at the University of Cologne, Germany, asked individuals with depression to talk about their experience of time, they described feeling that "everyone is passing me by" and "I am slower than everyone else." The most typical account, according to the researchers, was that "the passage of time turned into a dragging, inexorable, and viscous continuance." These words echo the slowing of time Bearden experienced in the Antelope Island 50K, where other runners passed him, one minute felt like ten, gravity seemed fifty times stronger, and it became nearly impossible to move forward. In a study of ultramarathoners competing in a 100-mile race, the runners reported "distortions in time . . . and a feeling that the race was 'never ending.'" Ultrarunner Robin Harvie remembers reaching the eighty-fifth mile of the Spartathalon in Greece, when "It was not just that I was slowing down; time itself seemed to have expanded, opening itself up to scrutiny at the atomic level." He describes the pain of the ultra-endurance athlete as "the agony of grief that words can no longer express." Learning to carry on in such a state is something that stays with you. Jennifer Pharr Davis, who in 2011 set the fastest known time for hiking the Appalachian Trail (46 days, 11 hours, and 20 minutes), writes in *The Pursuit of Endurance* that one of the most important things she's learned is, "You don't have to get rid of the pain to move forward. The hurt we experience in life might never fully go away; it could ebb and flow for an eternity. You can make progress and appreciate the times when life isn't as much of a struggle. And you can pray, and cry, and wrestle through the rest."

The strategies that ultra-endurance athletes use to withstand the lowest points of a race are a window into how humans endure hardship. Researcher Karen Weekes followed ten athletes at the Ironman World Championship in Monterrey, Mexico, as they attempted to complete ten triathlons in ten days—a total of 24 miles of swimming, 1,120 miles of biking, and 262 miles of running—to learn how they dealt with the pain, self-doubt, and exhaustion. Their answers, taken out of context, resemble a list one might generate by speaking to survivors of trauma or loss, or to patients undergoing difficult medical treatment, or to individuals struggling to stay sober. The athletes learned to focus on the present moment. They didn't let themselves get overwhelmed by thinking too far ahead. When the totality of what they faced overwhelmed them, they committed to finishing just one more lap, one more mile, or one more step.

To tap into positive emotions that could sustain them, they listened to music and replayed treasured memories in their minds. They gave themselves permission to cry, rage, or rest when they needed to. Almost all of the athletes took strength from thinking about loved ones. One found the will to keep going by recalling an email his youngest son had sent him, saying how proud he was of his dad. Another held entire conversations with family and friends in her mind. Two imagined being with deceased loved ones—a child and a husband—and found that this connection helped them tap into a reserve of energy that took them beyond their usual capacity to carry on. Several talked to God, praying, asking for support, and offering gratitude. Others found that they could overcome their pain and fatigue by dedicating their efforts to others, thinking about a loved one who was struggling or remembering the cause they were raising funds for by racing.

Many focused on the impermanence of their present pain. As one athlete told herself, "Sooner or later, the last lap will be done." This mentality wasn't simply about imagining a pain-free future. It was also about savoring a present moment that included both pleasure and pain. One athlete pretended that whatever lap he was swimming or mile he was biking was the last he would ever do in his life. This mindset brought out an anticipatory nostalgia and a fierce desire to enjoy the moment fully, even with the pain it contained.

To an outside observer, it might seem as though these psychological strategies are a means to an end, mental skills you need to perform the task of physical endurance. But when you listen to athletes, it's not at all clear that's how they perceive things. Many seem to take the reverse perspective: The physical hardship is the means to cultivating the mental strengths. When I spoke with Christina Torres, a thirty-year-old English teacher in Honolulu, Hawaii, about long-distance running, she mentioned the hymn "It Is Well with My Soul"—quite a departure from the songs runners commonly cite for inspiration, such as the themes from *Rocky* or *Chariots of Fire*. The lyrics were written in 1873 by Horatio Spafford shortly after the ocean liner his wife and children had been traveling on, the SS *Ville du Havre*, hit another ship and sank. His wife was rescued, unconscious, from the Atlantic Ocean, but all four of their daughters drowned. When Spafford got word by telegraph, he boarded a ship to meet his grieving wife in Europe. That ship's captain, aware of Spafford's loss, informed him when they reached the latitude and longitude where his children had drowned. There Spafford wrote the lines that would become a comfort to many: "When sorrows like sea billows roll; / Whatever my lot, Thou has taught me to say, / It is well, it is well, with my soul." With its message about maintaining faith in trying circumstances, the song is a popular choice at funerals.

This hymn may seem an odd reference for running, but for Torres, it expresses one of the main reasons she runs. "When I'm tired or a mile hurts, the beautiful thing running has taught me is it won't always hurt. In some way, it gets better. Joy cometh in the morning." When Torres runs, each step forward through discomfort and doubt is a practice of faith, a way of saying, *It is well with my soul*. "If God brings you to it, he will bring you through it. Running opened this up for me. It will be hard, it will hurt, but the struggle ends. Running made that visceral. The hill will finish." I heard similar sentiments from other athletes, who found in physical suffering a knowledge that landed deep in their bones. It is one thing to believe in something—in your capacity to survive, in the grace of God, or simply that this, too, shall pass. It is another thing to feel it in your body.

In 2016, Torres ran the Kauai Marathon. She describes the course as "a series of brutal, soul-crushing hills in some of the most beautiful places you've ever seen." At several points during the two-thousand-foot climb of the race course, Torres felt discouraged by her slower-than-expected pace and by seeing other runners pass her. But at mile eighteen, she reached the peak of a set of hills and the course opened up to a beautiful vista. As she looked out and took in the view, something inside her shifted, and she was overcome with a sense of gratitude. *What a gift it is to be able to run*, she thought. *How blessed am I*. She heard her grandfather's voice saying, "Appreciate this, *mija*." Torres started to cry, overwhelmed by joy. And as she ran downhill, she said over and over, "Thank you. Thank you."

Later, when I thought about this story, it occurred to me that almost all long-distance races take place outdoors. Other than the occasional fundraiser, people don't run ultramarathons on a treadmill. They roam wild terrain, follow the path of rivers, climb mountains, and descend through canyons. What separates even the most punishing ultra-endurance events from masochism is context. The events are not about suffering for suffering's sake, but suffering in a natural environment that invites, almost guarantees, moments of self-transcendence. If endurance training is in part about learning how to suffer well, it helps to put yourself in surroundings that inspire awe or gratitude. Outdoors, you can be stunned by a sudden change in landscape or enthralled by the appearance of wildlife. You can find yourself entranced by the stars at night or heartened by the first light of dawn. These transcendent emotions put personal pain and fatigue in a different context. It is impossible to understand what ultra-endurance athletes are doing without taking this into account. Experiencing a state of elevation during a moment of deep exhaustion provides a reminder that flashes of pure happiness can take you by surprise even when things seem the most bleak. Knowing this is possible is how we survive our worst pain. Finding a way for suffering and joy to coexist—that is how humans endure the seemingly unendurable.

• • •

At the annual Yukon Arctic Ultra, competitors from around the world attempt to follow the Yukon Quest trail across the Canadian Yukon Territory, covering three hundred miles on foot, cross-country ski, or mountain bike. The waiver that entrants sign forces them to acknowledge the possibility of dehydration, hypothermia, frostbite, avalanche, falling through thin ice, wild animal attacks, mental trauma, and serious physical injury, including death. During the 2018 race, temperatures fell to 49 below zero, and all but one competitor dropped out due to illness, exhaustion, or equipment failure. The organizers ended the event early, and South African runner Jethro De Decker was declared the winner when he reached a checkpoint at 3:45 A.M., thirty-two miles from the finish line.

One of the last athletes to exit the race, sixty-one-year-old

Roberto Zanda, was taken away by helicopter with frostbite so severe, he faced the amputation of both hands and both feet. Soon after, he gave an interview to the Canadian Broadcasting Corporation from his hospital bed in Whitehorse, Canada. His frostbitten hands and lower legs were wrapped in thick bandages, and he did not yet know if circulation would return. The sixty-one-year-old athlete—whose nickname, Massiccione, means "The Tough One"—told the CBC that "being alive is more important than hands and feet," and that he was looking forward to continuing to race, "even if it is with prosthetics." Six weeks later, unable to save his limbs, doctors amputated Zanda's right hand and both legs below the knee. He has since been fitted with carbon-fiber legs and a state-of-the-art bionic hand. He resumed training in his hometown of Cagliari, Sardinia. By summer, he had signed up to run his first race on new legs, a 155-mile ultramarathon across the deserts of Namibia.

When philosophy graduate student Kirsty-Ann Burroughs interviewed endurance runners about their race experiences, one theme that stood out was the importance of hope. "Each runner was responsible for allowing hope to get the better of despair," Burroughs writes. "Hope is what makes active endurance possible." The ability of ultra-endurance athletes to keep moving forward can be at once inspiring and bewildering. Watching a video of one of Roberto Zanda's first uphill hikes on carbon fiber legs—in which he comments, "I chose to live" and vows to run the same hill within two months—made me wonder: Are ultra-endurance athletes drawn to the sport because they possess an innate capacity to keep going? Or does the training itself produce their remarkable hardiness? The answer is surely a mixture of both. However, new research gives reason to believe that resilience is an outcome, not just a necessary precursor, of endurance.

In 2015, scientists from the Center for Space Medicine and Extreme Environments in Berlin followed athletes competing in the Yukon Arctic Ultra. They wanted to know: How does the human body cope in such a brutal context? When the researchers analyzed the hormones in the bloodstreams of the athletes, one hormone, irisin, was wildly elevated. Irisin is best known for its role in metabolism—it helps the body burn fat as fuel. But irisin also has powerful effects on the brain. Irisin stimulates the brain's reward system, and the hormone may be a natural antidepressant. Lower levels are associated with an increased risk of depression, and elevated levels can boost motivation and enhance learning. Injecting the protein directly into the brains of mice—not something scientists are ready to try with humans—reduces behaviors associated with depression, including learned helplessness and immobility in the face of threats. Higher blood levels of irisin are also associated with superior cognitive functioning, and may even prevent neurodegenerative diseases such as Alzheimer's.

The Yukon Arctic Ultra athletes entered the event with extraordinarily high blood levels of this hormone, far beyond levels seen in most humans. Over the course of the event, their irisin levels climbed higher. Even as their bodies fell victim to hypothermia and exhaustion, the athletes were bathing their brains in a chemical that preserves brain health and prevents depression. Why were their blood levels of irisin so elevated? The answer lies in both the nature of the event and what the athletes had to do to get there. Irisin has been dubbed the "exercise hormone," and it is the best-known example of a *myokine,* a protein that is manufactured in your muscles and released into your bloodstream during physical activity. (*Myo* means muscle, and *kine* means "set into motion by.") One of the greatest recent scientific breakthroughs in human biology is the realization that skeletal muscles act as an endocrine organ. Your muscles, like your adrenal and pituitary glands, secrete proteins that affect every system of your body. One of these proteins is irisin. Following a single treadmill workout, blood levels of irisin increase by 35 percent. The Yukon Arctic Ultra required up to fifteen hours a day of exercise. Muscle shivering—a form of muscle contraction—also triggers the release of irisin into the bloodstream. For the Yukon Arctic Ultra competitors, the combination of extreme environment and extreme exertion led to exceptionally high levels of this myokine.

Irisin is not the only beneficial myokine your muscles dispatch into your bloodstream when you exercise. A 2018 scientific paper identified thirty-five proteins released by your quadriceps during a single hour of bicycling. Some of these myokines help your muscles grow stronger, while others regulate blood sugar, reduce inflammation, or even kill cancer cells. Scientists now believe that many of the long-term health benefits of exercise are due to the beneficial myokines released during muscle contraction.

While much of the research on myokines has focused on how these chemicals prevent disease, some of their most potent effects are on mental health. For example, vascular endothelial growth factor and brain-derived neurotrophic factor (originally named this because scientists thought it was produced only in the brain), protect the health of brain cells, and even help the brain generate new neurons. Every known effective biological treatment for depression, including medications and electroshock therapy, also increases levels of these neurotrophins.

Another myokine, glial-derived neurotrophic factor, protects dopamine neurons in the midbrain. The destruction of dopamine neurons contributes to a wide range of disorders, including depression and Parkinson's disease, and is one of the most insidious side effects of drug addiction. By releasing a neurotrophic factor that preserves dopamine neurons, exercise may prevent, slow, or even reverse these conditions. Still other myokines decrease inflammation in the brain, which can also prevent neurological disorders and reduce symptoms of depression and anxiety. Some myokines even metabolize a neurotoxic chemical caused by chronic stress, turning it into a harmless substance in your bloodstream before it can reach the brain. You can't see or feel this alchemy as it occurs, but it takes place every time you exercise.

One of the first scientific papers to write about exercise-induced myokines labeled them "hope molecules." Ultra-endurance athletes talk about the metaphor of putting one foot in front of the other—how learning that you *can* take one more step, even when it feels like you can't possibly keep going, builds confidence and courage. The existence of hope molecules reveals that this is not merely a metaphor. Hope can begin in your muscles. Every time you take a single step, you contract over two hundred myokine-releasing muscles. The very same muscles that propel your body forward also send proteins to your brain that stimulate the neurochemistry of resilience. Importantly, you don't need to run an ultramarathon across the Arctic to infuse your bloodstream with these chemicals. Any movement that involves muscular contraction—which is to say, all movement—releases beneficial myokines.

It seems likely that some ultra-endurance athletes are drawn to the sport precisely because they have a natural capacity to endure. The extreme circumstances of these events allow them to both challenge and enjoy that part of their personality. Yet it's also possible that the intense physical training contributes to the mental toughness that ultra-endurance athletes demonstrate. Endurance activities like walking, hiking, jogging, running, cycling, and swimming, as well as high-intensity exercise such as interval training, are especially likely to produce a myokinome that supports mental health. Among those who are already active, increasing training intensity or volume—going harder, faster, further, or longer—can jolt muscles to stimulate an even greater myokine release. In one study, running to exhaustion increased irisin levels for the duration of the run and well into a recovery period—an effect that could be viewed as an intravenous dose of hope. Many of the world's top ultra-endurance athletes have a history of depression, anxiety, trauma, or addiction. Some, like ultrarunner Shawn Bearden, credit the sport with helping to save their lives. This, too, is part of what draws people to the ultra-endurance world. You can start off with seemingly superhuman abilities to endure, or you can build your capacity for resilience one step at a time.

Months after I spoke with Bearden, an image from his Instagram account appeared in my feed. It was taken from the middle of a paved road that stretches toward a mountain range, with grassy fields on either side. The sky is blue, except for a huge dark cloud that appears to be hovering directly over the person taking the photo. I remembered how Bearden had described his depression as a black thundercloud rolling in. Under the Instagram photo, Bearden had written, "Tons of wind today, making an easy run far more challenging. So happy to be able to do this. Every day above ground is a good day." Below, a single comment cheered him on, like a fellow runner on the trail: "Amen to this! Keep striving."

...

At age fifty-seven, adventure athlete Terri Schneider has summited the highest peaks of Africa, South America, and Europe. She has run the Sahara Desert, biked the mountains of Bhutan during monsoon season, and trekked with the Achuar in the Amazon rain forest of Ecuador. The highlights reel of Schneider's career could easily be mistaken for a surrealist nightmare. While running the Gobi Desert's salt flats in China, she found herself plunged thigh-deep in mud, her shoes sucked off her feet as if by some hungry subterranean creature. (She ran the rest of the race in socks.) Mountain biking down a 10,000-foot volcano in Costa Rica, she crashed on the rocks, and, while splayed on the ground trying to recover, was attacked by a stray dog. She has been thrown out of a paddleboat into shark- and sea-snake-infested waters. She has gotten stuck in quicksand on horseback. During one jungle trek, leeches attracted by her body heat flung themselves at her from the darkness and crawled into her gloves, up her pant legs, and into any opening they could find; she recalls watching her own blood seep out of the eyelets of her shoes and the stitches of her clothing.

These are not the stories Schneider tells when you ask her, "What are the worst things you've experienced during an event?" These are the stories she tells when trying to explain what makes being an ultra-endurance athlete worthwhile. Her adventures play out in some of the most stunning locations in the world, places most people will never get to experience. "To be a human in those environments, you're required to physically suffer in a lot of ways," Schneider told me. The juxtaposition between the beauty around her and what she had to endure to get there is deeply satisfying. "I can pause for a moment within the suffering and look around, and go, because I'm suffering, I'm here right now, and that's amazing. I'm here because I toiled to arrive. It's a testament to what's possible for the human mind and body."

When I asked Schneider how she ended up a professional adventure athlete, she explained, "I was never abused. I never had an eating disorder, no major trauma other than average-Joe getting my heart broken. My story is just becoming a strong woman." She remembers the first time she felt the sheer pleasure of pushing her body's limits. She was ten years old and running in a cross-country meet. She came in second to last but didn't care. "Pushing my body, this whole new world opened up to me. It felt joyful. It was interesting and unique and exciting. Even after all these years, I feel gratitude that I can still go out and push my body and have that sort of feeling." When Schneider was young, her mother warned her that if she ran too much, her uterus would fall out—something she claimed to have learned from *Reader's Digest*. During her adventures, Schneider feels liberated from expectations about how a woman should think or behave. "Doing something physically difficult in nature, as a woman, it's not like anything else you do in life," she told me. "There are no social reference points, no cultural messaging, no visuals requiring me to be or think of myself in a certain way. Nature wipes that clean." She likes who she becomes in the unpredictable wilderness, away from the pressure of social norms. "It's the same Terri I always am, but it's decisive Terri, strong Terri, confident Terri, content Terri, and grateful Terri."

When choosing adventures, Schneider seeks out what she calls the "big stretches"—events that require her to go beyond what she has done before and beyond what she is certain she can do. Hers is not just a curiosity about whether she can accomplish something, but also about how the experience will unfold and how she will respond in a new and challenging environment. She wants to test the limits of what is possible to see what it brings out in her. This is a common motivation among adventure athletes. As Jethro De Decker said after surviving the catastrophic 2018 Yukon Arctic Ultra, "Can there be a better way to work out who you are?"

One of Schneider's most memorable big stretches took place almost twenty-five years ago, in the very first Eco-Challenge, a ten-day nonstop team adventure race in Utah. The five-member teams would attempt to cover 376 miles on horseback, foot, and mountain bikes, while also scaling rocks, rappelling into canyons, and navigating the wild rivers in rafts and canoes. Fifty teams of experienced athletes entered the challenge, but only twenty-one completed it. (A medical journal later described the race as a case study in "unprecedented and significant" physical risks, even by the standard of ultra-endurance competitions.) When Schneider signed up for the event, she had less experience rock-climbing than in the other skills, and she still had a tendency to panic when she looked down. In practice climbs that required her to rappel only thirty feet, she found herself frozen with fear—a feeling she describes as being immobilized by an evil spirit. Part of what drew her to the Eco-Challenge was knowing that she would have to work through this fear.

The biggest climb in the race was straight up a 1,200-foot cliff on fixed ropes. Every 100 feet, she would have to stop on the cliff face and transfer to a new rope. If she made a single mistake, she would free-fall into the river below. When Schneider's team reached the climb, she stood at the base of the cliff, paralyzed. In her memoir, *Dirty Inspirations*, she recalls considering her options: quit; climb the cliff while feeling like a hostage to her fright; or accept the fear, and take the 1,200-foot climb one arm reach at time. Schneider chose the last option. As she climbed, the fear ascended with her. To stay calm, Schneider focused on two sensations: her hand touching the rock and the sound of the rope sliding through the ascender attached to her harness. It took her four hours to reach the top of the cliff. Standing at the edge, she looked down to savor the magnificent view. "What it taught me wasn't that you overcome fear or make fear go away," Schneider told me. "What changed for me is I can have a relationship with fear where I'm holding the cards. I can control how I experience fear. I learned I can analyze my fear, look at it, create a relationship with it, have it be information rather than a showstopper. I can be the decider."

I know firsthand the terror Schneider experienced while climbing, although on a much smaller scale. Years ago, I tried indoor rock-climbing with my husband. Agreeing to this was, for me, a big stretch. Just standing near a window in a tall building triggers vertigo and the sensation that I am already falling. At the climbing gym, making my way up the artificial rock formation, I was strapped into a harness. My safety rope was controlled by my husband, who would break my fall if I slipped. And yet I found that despite these safety mechanisms, I could not climb higher than a very specific elevation. Around twenty feet up, my body froze, and my brain said, *Get me down NOW*. It didn't matter what wall I was climbing, or what configuration the hand- and footholds were in. The neurons in my motor cortex could not or would not command my arm to reach for the next handhold; the fear circuit deep in my midbrain held them captive.

At the time, I assumed that my twenty-foot psychological ceiling was unbreakable, some biological safety mechanism inherited from risk-averse ancestors. I never found out what would happen if I tried to climb above that mental barrier. Months after talking with Schneider, I found myself thinking about her on the cliff face, scaling 1,200 feet one hand-reach at a time. Her accomplishment seemed so far outside what I could imagine myself doing. Yet the way she described fear was so familiar. I told my husband we were going back to Planet Granite, the climbing gym where I had hit my fear ceiling fifteen years earlier.

After a one-hour safety class, I was once again strapped into a harness attached to a rope that hung fifty feet from the top of the wall. My husband held the rope, ready to pull the slack as I climbed and prepared to catch me if I fell. Next to me, two parents were coaching a young boy—maybe ten years old—up the wall, and I found myself climbing parallel to him. The desire to stop kicked in soon, after I had made only a few moves. I wasn't anywhere near my previous best of twenty feet off the floor. But the boy climbing next to me was clearly having so much fun, and I felt myself pulled up somehow by his enthusiasm. As I got higher on the wall, the instinct to stop got stronger. I thought about Terri Schneider and how she must have felt at the 600-foot mark of her big climb. I said to myself, *Just make the next move, just keep climbing.* It helped that I could physically sense the support of my husband through the tension he maintained in my rope, his way of letting me know, "I've got you." More than once, I felt an encouraging tug on the rope, as if he was trying to lift me up.

I made it up the wall on my first try, something I hadn't planned for. I had expected to fail, so strong was my belief in my own fear. When I got to the top, I clanged the cowbell that was anchored to the wall so climbers could signal their success. As my hand touched the metal, I realized that I had never once imagined this part of the outing. I had pictured arriving, strapping myself in the harness, and even making it off the ground. But no part of me had bothered to mentally preview something I hadn't thought was possible. Once I was back on the ground, I felt the shock of what I had done. My husband said, "You did it!" I was too stunned to say much in return. After my first successful climb, I immediately scaled two more routes to the top of the wall, to make sure it hadn't been a fluke. My fear never fully disappeared, but something else—a sense of determination, even fun—joined it on the ride up.

I'd been carrying a story in my head for fifteen years that my brain wouldn't let me climb higher than twenty feet. What had changed? As far as I could tell, what made the most difference was talking to Schneider. At first I was just inspired, thinking, *Wow, that could never be me.* But then somehow her story opened the possibility that the same bravery was available to me. While I was climbing, being able to literally sense my husband's support kept me going when fear threatened to paralyze me. The ten-year-old boy climbing next to me, with his unbridled excitement, deserves credit, too. His joy was contagious.

When I headed to Planet Granite, I knew that I wanted to make room for fear, courage, and joy to coexist on the climb. It wasn't until I was on the wall, climbing, that I realized other people can hold the courage and joy for you until you can find your own. I didn't have to generate every ounce of what I needed by myself. I could expand my idea of what the container of my experience was—make it big enough to include those who had gone before me and those who were sharing it with me, even on the periphery.

When I spoke with Schneider, she told me that after a big stretch, "you walk away from the experience, look back over your shoulder, and think, *Oh, wow, look at what I did.* Knowing that you did it never leaves you. No matter what comes later in life, that thing will always be with you, something you did." After my climb, I felt this self-confidence. I must have said, "I did it!" at least a half-dozen times at the gym and on the car ride home. But later, as I reflected on the experience, what I felt even more was appreciation. Maybe one of the gifts of a big stretch is that you can choose the lesson you take from it. You get to polish the memory that stays with you. Schneider had told me how thrilling it was for her to do solo adventures, to disappear into the wild and discover that she could survive on her own. For me, the lesson that I most wanted to carry forward, the memory I had already started to look back on with wonder, was the opposite. That when I faced a wall I was afraid to climb, I found the support I needed. After that big stretch, it became easier to imagine something I had never really let myself believe. Not just that I could ring a cowbell fifty feet off the ground, but something even more reassuring. That when I found myself in a situation I didn't know how to get through on my own, an assemblage of family, friends, and even strangers might rally around me.

···

One of the most celebrated moments of Olympic history took place at the 1992 games in Barcelona, when British runner and world-record holder Derek Redmond finished the 400-meter semifinals dead last. An injury had kept him from competing in the 1988 games in Seoul, and Barcelona was widely considered his opportunity to medal. If you watch a video of the event, here's what you'll see: Redmond starts strong, but fifteen seconds into the race, he clutches his right leg and slows to a hop. Two seconds later, he collapses onto the track. His first thought, he later explained, was that he had been shot in the back of his thigh. In reality, the violent pain was his hamstring muscle snapping off the bone.

By the time Redmond is able to stand back up, every one of his competitors has crossed the finish line. The race is over. Yet Redmond refuses to quit. He begins to hop awkwardly on one leg, grimacing as he breaks away from the television cameras and medics that have swarmed to the spot where he collapsed. Meanwhile, a middle-aged man wearing a baseball cap has sprung from his seat in the stadium and is rushing the track. Officials try to block the man, but he pushes past them. The man reaches Redmond and places a hand on the back of his shoulder. Redmond starts to shake it off, thinking it is another race official trying to stop him. Then he hears, "Derek, it's me." Redmond turns to see that it is his father.

Redmond's father grabs his hand and wraps an arm around Redmond's waist. He jogs alongside his son until Redmond begins to wail and slows to a walk. As they take halting steps, Redmond buries his face in his father's chest. "You can stop now," his father tells him. "You haven't got nothing to prove." Redmond insists, "Get me back into lane five. I want to finish." The two continue to walk. A white-shirted Olympic official tries to stop them, but Redmond's father brushes him off and shouts, "I'm his father, leave him alone!" Cameramen surround them. When Redmond covers his face in shame, his father grabs his wrist and pulls his hand down. The crowd begins to cheer, and Redmond and his father finish the last hundred meters together.

After the event, a Canadian competitor sent Redmond a note, calling Redmond's finish "the purest, most courageous example of grit and determination I have seen." Redmond's desire to keep going and his ability to persevere through his pain are indeed remarkable. Yet I don't think it's his persistence that people are most moved by. It's his father, the person who didn't belong on the track, who wasn't an athlete, but whose body sprang into action to help his son. It's also the sight of someone so strong, a national sports hero, accepting that support. This Olympic moment touches us—people weep watching the video—not just because Redmond persisted, but because it demonstrates how much we depend on one another to keep going.

When you listen to the stories of ultra-endurance athletes, one of the first things you realize is that no one is doing it all by themselves. While an athlete's initial motivation is often competitive—a desire to prove themselves, or to do something that "ordinary" people can't—they experience a more complex reality during the events. Surviving an ultra-endurance race highlights not only their individual strength but also their reliance on others. Many athletes take heart simply knowing that there are others struggling through the same event. One runner told me that when he finds himself alone on the course, with no one else in sight, he likes to think of the other participants who are also out there somewhere, facing their own demons. As another ultrarunner explains, "Things seem easier when they're shared among more people." Most athletes have support teams—friends, family, coaches—who help them prepare for and get through big events. Volunteers staff aid stations along the route, helping race participants refuel, lance blisters, or summon the will to continue. The athletes also help one another, sharing personal supplies or sacrificing their best time to make sure that a fellow competitor can keep going. When software engineer Joy Ebertz was felled by gastrointestinal problems in the middle of a fifty-mile race, she found herself dehydrated and five long miles from the next aid station. Another runner passing her stopped to assist. "He gave me his water and walked with me to the next aid station, completely ruining the time he would have gotten in that race." During one ultrarunner's first overnight 62-mile trail race, he became stranded and alone in the dark when the battery of his headlamp ran out. The next runner who arrived ran with him, illuminating the path for both of them until dawn broke. As one runner explains, "If you have socks in your pocket and someone needs socks, you've just lost a pair of socks . . . and that's okay, these things all work out in the end. It really does mean that you're part of the community, you're part of the family."

When researcher Jenna Quicke asked ultrarunners to choose a photo of something that represented ultrarunning to them, they didn't submit photos of sneakers or bloodied feet. Nor did they send snapshots of race medals or scenes of the outdoor environments they raced in. Most chose pictures of themselves with other runners. "Community was what was visible in these images," Quicke writes. Part of what bonds these athletes is the pain they endure. Sharing a physically painful experience—even something as simple as holding your hand in ice water, eating a hot chili pepper, or doing squats to exhaustion—increases trust and closeness among strangers. The bonds forged are much stronger when the pain is part of an event that holds personal meaning and is celebrated by others. Anthropologists Harvey Whitehouse and Jonathan A. Lanman write that collective rituals that include pain bond us to others by "hijacking our kinship psychology" and "fusing us to fellow ritual participants." In other words, when you go through an intense and difficult experience with others, you become family. As one participant in the famous fire-walking ritual of San Pedro Manrique told a researcher, "When you go up there, everyone is your brother." Another said, "The next day, you see another fire-walker in the street, and you know you've been through this together, you've bonded, you have a different relationship to this person."

In ultra-endurance events, the sense of kinship also derives from the physical intimacy of caring for others and being cared for. As I read accounts and watched footage of support crews, volunteers, and fellow competitors tending to bloody and blistered feet, offering a shoulder to lean or cry on, helping athletes stay hydrated after vomiting and diarrhea, I remembered something Niki Flemmer, a nurse practitioner who works with cancer patients, had told me. "When faced with an illness, so much of the bullshit is stripped away," she said. "When we are vulnerable, our capacity for connection, although perhaps harder to lean into, is deepened." No doubt this is part of what binds ultra-endurance athletes together, as the realities of the human body dispel any illusions of invincibility. According to a survey of hospice care nurses, one of the most common concerns at the end of life is not wanting to be a burden on others. Observing the rituals of care that take place during ultra-endurance events—the accepted, even welcomed physical intimacy of the tasks—I thought again of how deeply these events rehearse the practices of human interdependence.

THE RECOGNITION OF OUR interdependence is a commonly treasured takeaway from pushing the limits of what a human can endure. The Marathon Monks of Mount Hiei, Japan, are often described as spiritual athletes. They rise at midnight to run 18.8 miles through the forested mountain. The monks run in all seasons and all weather, including snow, with nothing but flimsy straw sandals to protect their feet. In heavy rain, they bring extra sandals for when their first pair disintegrates. The monks rest only once during the 18.8 miles, sitting to recite a two-minute prayer. Their daily runs are considered a spiritual practice much like studying ancient texts or sitting in silent meditation. The tradition dates to the period between 1310 and 1571, and since 1885, forty-six monks have fulfilled a vow to complete 1,000 runs in seven years. As they progress through their vows, the monks' nightly runs grow longer. By the end of their final year, they run 52.2 miles, the equivalent of two marathons, without rest.

Endo Mitsunaga is one of the few living Marathon Monks of Mount Hiei who has completed the full seven-year commitment. In 2010, he spoke with National Public Radio about the greatest spiritual lessons gained in his journey. He pointed to a nine-day sleepless fast that takes place after a monk has completed the first seven hundred runs. The ceremony left Mitsunaga so weak, he survived only by being cared for by fellow monks. The most lasting and meaningful insight from his epic seven-year cultivation of physical and mental endurance was this: "Everybody thinks they're living on their own without help from others. This is not possible."

The willingness to rely on others—for morale or physical support—can be a valuable lesson that extends beyond the race course. During Shawn Bearden's first 100-mile event, a distance that takes the average participant twenty-eight hours to finish, his running coach kept him company during the overnight part of the run. "I had this idea that I wanted to do it all myself, but under these conditions, I needed the support," he says. During the second half of the race, it would have been easy for Bearden to slip into not taking care of himself. His coach checked in, asking, "Are you drinking? Are you eating?" Accepting these nudges toward self-care can be a revolutionary act for someone who usually suffers in silence. It's a way to practice not pushing others away when they ask, "Are you okay?" or "What can I do?"

Bearden recognizes that his long-standing "go it alone, do it yourself" approach to life has been one of the triggers for his depression. He describes the mindset as "the sense of being alone, being responsible for living up to one hundred percent of my potential in every aspect, being the best I can be, and I have to do it all myself." Having his coach run alongside him—and not feeling like this was a crutch—was a revelation. "I was coming to appreciate that I was still doing it myself, but I had a friend there that I was sharing it with, and that didn't mean I was incapable," he told me. "Before, if something took any help, it would mean I was weak."

On a recent blog post, Bearden shared with his ultrarunning community that for most of his life, he was unable to imagine a future version of himself who was older than forty-five. He had always believed he would take his own life before he reached that age. In the post, Bearden reflects on how running has become both a form of therapy for him and a source of joy. He expresses gratitude to his wife for supporting him through his darkest moments and describes how accepting her help was one of the most difficult and important things he had ever done. He encourages anyone who is contemplating suicide or struggling with depression to know that they aren't alone, and not to be afraid to ask for help. The occasion of the blog post was his forty-sixth birthday. As he wrote, "There's no age I can't see beyond now."

FINAL THOUGHTS

While I was writing this book, I used a corkboard that runs from floor to ceiling in my home office. At first the board was sparsely filled with scribbled notes on index cards, the names of sources I planned to contact, and scientific abstracts I needed to follow up on. As the book progressed, many of the people I spoke with sent me photographs related to their stories. I printed them out and pinned them to the board, along with photos and screen captures of videos they had posted on social media.

One of my favorite photos on the corkboard was shared with me by Kimberly Sogge, a member of the eight-woman masters' crew at the Ottawa Rowing Club. It was taken in October 2017, when the crew competed in the fifty-third Head of the Charles Regatta, the world's largest two-day rowing event. Over one weekend, more than three hundred thousand spectators flock to the banks and bridges of the Charles River, which divides Boston from Cambridge, to watch athletes from around the world propel sculling and sweep-oared racing shells up the river. The Ottawa crew had won a lottery spot in the Women's Senior Masters race, in which the average age of rowers must be at least fifty. Participating in the regatta was a dream come true for the women. After the team arrived in Cambridge, the crew's coxswain, who steers the shell and coaches the rowers, gave each of the women a gift. Her eight-year-old daughter had cut hearts out of construction paper for the crew to take to the regatta. The young girl was enraptured with the Disney movie *Moana*, and she wanted the women to be able to carry the Heart of Te Fiti with them on the water.

The Women's Senior Masters race began just after ten A.M. on Saturday. The Ottawa crew had stuffed the construction-paper hearts down their matching red tank tops and into their sports bras, along with their IDs. The weather was unseasonably summerlike, the sun shining as the crew carried a fifty-eight-foot shell over their heads to the dock, then into the water, where hundreds of boats were slowly navigating toward the entrance point. The women took their seats facing the coxswain. Each handled a single oar sporting the blade of the Ottawa Rowing Club. As they rowed to the starting point, the coxswain said, "Ladies, we're here," reminding them to enjoy the moment. When the official called out, "Ottawa Rowing Club, Bow 30, you're up!," the coxswain yelled, "This is it! Let's do it!"

Rowers use their sense of hearing more than their vision, so what Sogge remembers most about the regatta are the sounds. The women's forceful exhalations, synchronized to each stroke. The oarlocks clicking together. The water rushing under the boat. The echo chamber created each time the boat went under a bridge. And the distinctive voice of a friend from Mexico City who stood on one of the bridges and screamed, "Go Ottawa!" when the crew passed by. As the shell made its way upriver, the crew relied on the trust and teamwork they had built in their training, at all the early-morning, after-work, and weekend practice sessions on the Ottawa River. As they approached the last hundred meters of the three-mile race, the coxswain called out, "Give it to me now, give me your hearts! I want the Heart of Te Fiti, and I want it now!"

"We rowed our hearts out," Sogge told me. "That was a moment of pain, hard work, mastery, and oneness that none of us will ever forget." The crew crossed the finish in twenty minutes and thirty-seven seconds, coming in thirty-first out of thirty-eight teams. They were thrilled with the results; they had achieved their goal of working together to complete an excellent technical race. As the crew paddled back to the dock, they paused and let the boat glide for a moment. The coxswain reminded the rowers of her daughter's gift. "Now you have to give your hearts to the river," she commanded. Exhausted and happy, the women pulled the now sweat-stained paper hearts out of their sports bras. On the count of three, they threw the hearts into the water. This is the photograph Sogge shared with me. It captures the exact moment the women stretched their arms to the sky. The gesture—their right arms raised, paper hearts clasped between thumbs and fingertips—is as synchronized as a rowing stroke. Sogge remembers feeling a sense of joy and letting go as the paper hearts fluttered away, thinking, *Even this beautiful thing is already water under the bridge.*

One day, as I glanced up at the corkboard in my home office for what must have been the hundredth time, I started to think about how interesting it was that these images existed. We don't document things that don't matter. These photos were captured because people were recording a moment they wanted to remember. It means something that people take and share videos of physical accomplishments, and that they fling sweaty arms around one another for a group selfie after a workout. And it means something that people cherish the mementos in these photos—that they display race bibs alongside family pictures, or hold on to T-shirts from twenty years ago. All of the images on the corkboard were evidence of how physical activity can bring people together and bring out the best in us. They were reminders of how even simple actions—lifting a heavy weight, scaling a wall, joining hands in a circle—can take on meaning in surprising ways. These moments get captured in photos, preserved through objects, and retold as stories. Memories crystallize around such moments of joy, connection, or triumph. And over time, identities are forged and communities formed.

In a 2017 essay, Norwegian ethicist Sigmund Loland posed the question: If it becomes possible, should we replace exercise with a pill? Scientists are already trying to manufacture medicines that mimic the health benefits of exercise. What if they succeed? "Considering exercise takes time and energy and usually financial resources in addition to implying a risk for injury, the only reason for not replacing exercise with a pill must be related to values in the very activity of exercising in itself," Loland writes. "Does exercise have such values, and if so, what are they?"

Based on what I've learned from the science and stories that fill this book and from my own direct experience, I would say the answer is a resounding yes. Movement offers us pleasure, identity, belonging, and hope. It puts us in places that are good for us, whether that's outdoors in nature, in an environment that challenges us, or with a supportive community. It allows us to redefine ourselves and reimagine what is possible. It makes social connection easier and self-transcendence possible. Each of these benefits can be realized through other means. There are multiple paths to self-discovery and many ways to build community. Happiness can be found in any number of roles and pastimes; solace can be taken in poetry, prayer, or art. Exercise need not replace any of these other sources of meaning and joy. Yet physical activity stands out in its ability to fulfill so many human needs, and that makes it worth considering as a fundamentally valuable endeavor. It is as if what is good in us is most easily activated by or accessed through movement. As rower Kimberly Sogge put it, when she described to me why the Head of the Charles Regatta was such a peak experience, "The highest spirit of humanity gets to come out." Ethicist Sigmund Loland came to a similar conclusion, declaring that an exercise pill would be a poor substitute for physical activity. As he wrote, "Rejecting exercise means rejecting significant experiences of being human."

Physical activity helps us tap into instincts that have allowed humans to survive for millennia: the abilities to persist, cooperate, and form communities of mutual support; to invest in the future, overcome obstacles, and endure hardships; to defend and protect the vulnerable; to sense ourselves connected to other people and the world we live in; to give back, reach out, and pull one another up. And the mechanism by which movement seems to accomplish all of this is *joy*. Joy is what ties together the neurochemistry of the runner's high, the elation of moving in synchrony, and the unity sensation in nature. It's what draws us to ritual and music, and what makes achieving a personal best, cooperating with others, and witnessing someone else's triumph so satisfying. When movement brings out the best in us, it does so by making us happy. Not only through short-lived feelings of pleasure or pride, but also in the deepest sense of the word. The happiness that comes from having a sense of purpose and from belonging. The happiness of feeling connected to something bigger than yourself. The happiness that is best described as hope.

It's not difficult to experience the psychological and social benefits of movement. As philosopher Doug Anderson writes, "the possibilities—the transformative traits of movement—are there for each of us if we will awaken to them, if we will pay attention to our own experiences." There's no training formula you have to follow. There is no one path or prescription except to follow your own joy. If you're looking for a guideline, it's this: Move. Any kind, any amount, and any way that makes you happy. Move whatever parts of your body still move, with gratitude. Move by yourself, and in community. Move in your home. Move outdoors. Move to music or in silence. Set goals that are personally meaningful. Take baby steps, then conquer a big stretch. Seek out new experiences and explore new identities. Pay attention to how activities make you feel and how they change you. Listen to your body. Give yourself permission to do what feels good. Revel in metaphor and meaning. Look for places, people, and communities that inspire you and make you feel welcomed. Keep following the thread of joy as long as you can.

As I was finishing revisions on this book, I added another photograph to my corkboard. It was taken after a dance class I taught at a local gym on Halloween. Despite the fact that the class took place at eight A.M., half of the participants arrived in costumes: a spider in its web, a black cat, a wizard, a bumblebee, a skeleton, and two Wonder Women. I had brought persimmons and harvest-crisp apples in a trick-or-treat bucket for everyone to enjoy after class. One of the other dancers brought chocolates. The playlist was mostly our standard songs, but I threw in a few Halloween surprises. We howled like wolves, lurched like zombies, and laughed at our own silliness.

Among the participants in class that day, one was undergoing chemotherapy, and another was grieving the recent loss of her husband. Another woman was recovering from both a traumatic brain injury and the death of her father. And yet they each found a reason to show up and dance—or perhaps, these were the reasons. After our cooldown stretch, as the next class was clamoring to get into the studio, we held them off so we could take a group photo. A couple of weeks later, one of the women in that photo sent me a note explaining what the class had meant to her over the past year. "Sometimes it's given me the opportunity to feel strong and empowered, sometimes to work through difficult emotions, and sometimes to feel joyful and optimistic. I had experienced these benefits before, but new this year was feeling really seen and supported by my wonderful classmates. Some of them were experiencing their own challenges, but by dancing together in community, I think we drew strength from each other, and I was reminded that I wasn't alone."

I printed out her email and pinned it on the corkboard, alongside the Halloween class photo, where they joined all the other moments captured by the people who had spoken with me for this book. There was Cathy Merrifield jumping into the water at Tough Mudder. A pack of GoodGym runners posing outside a food bank where they had just sorted donations. CrossFit coach Reverend Katie Norris carrying her husband on her back along the beach. The "We Are Family" T-shirt Costas Karageorghis made for his track team at Brunel University. Jody Bender running her first 5K on the treadmill at physical therapy. Green Gym Camden volunteers celebrating the group's ten-year anniversary of caring for green spaces in their community. Ultrarunner Shawn Bearden's Instagram snapshot from the open road. Joanna Bonilla boxing with Devon Palermo at DPI Adaptive Fitness, earning her place on the Wall of Greatness. The Dance for PD dancers in the rehearsal room at Juilliard, their arms lifted in the air in a gesture of joy. The rack of half-marathon race medals in Nora Haefele's living room. Amara MacPhee posing with her 305 Fitness "fit fam" at her first class after having open heart surgery. My sister and her husband running a race side by side, pushing their twin girls in strollers. My eight A.M. dance class, taking the opportunity to celebrate life with friends.

As I stood at the corkboard, looking at all those images of persistence, bravery, and community, my heart swelled. *This is what hope looks like.*

This book includes the personal stories of many individuals. When these individuals are identified by their full names, it is because I received permission to share their stories and to include their full names, or because their stories had been previously published or shared publicly. When a person is identified by a first name only, it is because the individual was willing to share a story but did not want to be identified (in which case, I gave them a pseudonym or used their true first name with permission), or because I could not reach that person to receive permission to share the story (for example, if the story comes from a case report in a scientific journal, and the individual was given a pseudonym by researchers). All quotes from named sources were obtained during personal interviews (in person or via phone, Skype, email, or social media), unless otherwise noted in the research references at the end of the book. The scientific references listed are representative sources supporting statements made in the book, but are not exhaustive. I have tried to include citations that will direct the reader to both important research reviews as well as any specific studies mentioned in the text. In this book, I describe research conducted on nonhuman animals. I believe that there are serious ethical considerations when it comes to both conducting and profiting from such studies. I have chosen to discuss animal studies when they represent a substantial part of the scientific basis for the idea I am explaining. These studies followed the scientific community's consensus for the ethical treatment of nonhuman subjects at the time they were conducted.

ACKNOWLEDGMENTS

Writing a book is its own kind of ultramarathon, and like any endurance athlete, I could not have reached the finish line alone.

On the publishing side, I owe so much to my agent, Ted Weinstein, who continues to be an incredible advocate and ally. Deep gratitude also goes to the entire team at Avery and Penguin Random House. To my publisher and editor, Megan Newman, thank you for taking on this project. You challenged me to think bigger, trust my curiosity, and follow the most fascinating threads. Thank you also to editor Nina Shield for your patience and guidance through the revision process, and to Hannah Steigmeyer for all the behind-the-scenes support. To Nancy Inglis and Janice Kurzius, thank you for not only catching errors but also elevating the manuscript. And to Lindsay Gordon and Casey Maloney, thank you for always making the publicity process fun. I'm so glad we've had the chance to keep working together over the years.

My family started supporting this book before they had any idea I would become an exercise instructor or an author. Thank you to my mother, Judith, for bringing home all those garage sale workout videos, and for putting me in musical theater and dance classes. Thank you to my father, Kevin, for driving me to and from all those classes and rehearsals. And to both my parents, thank you for demonstrating—and passing on—a devotion to teaching. To my twin sister, Jane, thank you for your encouragement in all things in life, and for your enthusiasm for the topic of this book in particular. It kept me motivated even when I didn't know how to move forward. To my husband, Brian, thank you for being a constant companion in this ultramarathon of a writing process. Like any good pacer, you provided moral support, kept me focused during the homestretch, and when I was exhausted and overwhelmed, reminded me why I was doing this.

I am thrilled to also have a chance to publicly thank some of the exercise and dance instructors who have contributed so much to my happiness and mental health over the years. There are more than I can name, but they include Barry Moore, Gerry Barney, and Linda Polvere, who nurtured my love of dance when I was young; the instructors at HealthWorks in Boston on Commonwealth Avenue, where I took my first kickboxing classes; the faculty of the dance department at Stanford University; Judi Sheppard Missett, Margaret Richards, and all the other pioneers and role models who have inspired me, including Nia founders Debbie Rosas and Carlos Rosas and the wonderful Nia trainers I've learned from; the fabulous Zumba educational specialists and jammers I've had the chance to dance with; the program directors and international presenting team of Les Mills; and the creators of all the programs that bring so many people joy, including BollyX, REFIT, and 305 Fitness.

A special thank-you to the communities where I've taught group exercise over the years, especially Stanford Aerobics and Yoga, where I led my first class in 2000 and continue to teach; and to Sarah Ramirez, my first Nia teacher, my favorite collaborator in spreading the joy of movement, and an individual who truly embodies what it means to build community and choose hope in the face of obstacles.

Most of all, I want to acknowledge the individuals who shared their personal stories in this book, and the organizations that allowed me to write about them. Thank you for your generosity. You took the time to participate in this project because you wanted to help and encourage others. Nothing could be closer to the heart of this book, and why I wrote it. I hope that you feel I captured something true and meaningful about your journey and what you bring to the world. And if this book makes a difference in the lives of others, your contribution will be one of the reasons why.

NOTES

Introduction

5 **As neuroscientist Daniel Wolpert writes:** Daniel M. Wolpert, Zoubin Ghahramani, and J. Randall Flanagan, "Perspectives and Problems in Motor Learning." *Trends in Cognitive Sciences* 5, no. 11 (2001): 487–94.

7 **As philosopher Doug Anderson observed:** Doug Anderson, "Recovering Humanity: Movement, Sport, and Nature." *Journal of the Philosophy of Sport* 28, no. 2 (2001): 140–50.

Chapter 1: The Persistence High

9 **In 1855, Scottish philosopher Alexander Bain:** Alexander Bain, *The Senses and the Intellect* (London: John W. Parker & Son, 1855).

9 **In his memoir *Footnotes*, cultural historian Vybarr Cregan-Reid:** Vybarr Cregan-Reid, *Footnotes: How Running Makes Us Human* (New York: Thomas Dunne Books/St. Martin's Press, 2017). Quote about the runner's high on p. 100.

9 **Trail runner and triathlete Scott Dunlap sums up:** Scott Dunlap, "Understanding the Runner's High." January 8, 2005; http://www .atrailrunnersblog.com/2005/01/understanding-runners-high.html.

9–10 **In *The Runner's High*, Dan Sturn describes:** Dan Sturn, "How Humans Fly." In Garth Battista, ed., *The Runner's High: Illumination and Ecstasy in Motion* (Halcottsville, NY: Breakaway Books, 2014). Quote appears on p. 178.

10 **On a Reddit forum dedicated to explaining:** https://www.reddit.com/r /running/comments/1nbmjc/what_does_the_runners_high_actually _feel_like/.

10 **Ultrarunner Stephanie Case describes her midrun glow:** Stephanie Case, "Riding the Runner's Highs and Braving the Lows." March 10, 2011; https://ultrarunnergirl.com/2011/03/10/highs_and_lows/.

10 **As biologist Dennis Bramble and paleoanthropologist Daniel Lieberman write:** Dennis M. Bramble and Daniel E. Lieberman, "Endurance Running and the Evolution of *Homo*." *Nature* 432, no. 7015 (2004): 345–52.

12 **"Nothing makes you feel less adequate as a man," Pontzer recalls:** Although Herman Pontzer shared this story with me in our conversation, the quote I used is from the Story Collider podcast where I first heard him tell it. You can listen to the story here: https://www .storycollider.org/stories/2016/10/22/herman-pontzer-burning-calories.

12 **As part of Pontzer's research project:** David A. Raichlen et al.,
    "Physical Activity Patterns and Biomarkers of Cardiovascular Disease
    Risk in Hunter-Gatherers." *American Journal of Human Biology* 29, no. 2
    (2017): doi: 10.1002/ajhb.22919.

13 **Contrast this to the United States:** Jared M. Tucker, Gregory J. Welk,
    and Nicholas K. Beyler, "Physical Activity in US Adults: Compliance
    with the Physical Activity Guidelines for Americans." *American Journal
    of Preventive Medicine* 40, no. 4 (2011): 454–61; Vijay R. Varma et al.,
    "Re-evaluating the Effect of Age on Physical Activity over the
    Lifespan." *Preventive Medicine* 101 (2017): 102–8.

13 **the Hadza show no signs of the cardiovascular disease:** Raichlen
    et al., "Physical Activity Patterns and Biomarkers of Cardiovascular
    Disease Risk in Hunter-Gatherers."

13 **physical activity . . . is correlated with a sense of purpose:** Stephanie
    A. Hooker and Kevin S. Masters, "Purpose in Life Is Associated with
    Physical Activity Measured by Accelerometer." *Journal of Health
    Psychology* 21, no. 6 (2016): 962–71.

13 **people are happier . . . when they are physically active:** Neal Lathia et al.,
    "Happier People Live More Active Lives: Using Smartphones to Link
    Happiness and Physical Activity." *PLOS ONE* 12, no. 1 (2017): e0160589.

13 **on days when people are more active:** Jaclyn P. Maher et al., "Daily
    Satisfaction with Life Is Regulated by Both Physical Activity and
    Sedentary Behavior." *Journal of Sport and Exercise Psychology* 36, no. 2
    (2014): 166–78.

14 **Regular exercisers who replace physical activity:** Romano Endrighi,
    Andrew Steptoe, and Mark Hamer, "The Effect of Experimentally
    Induced Sedentariness on Mood and Psychobiological Responses to
    Mental Stress." *The British Journal of Psychiatry: The Journal of Mental
    Science* 208, no. 3 (2016): 245–51.

14 **When adults are randomly assigned to reduce their daily step count:**
    Meghan K. Edwards and Paul D. Loprinzi, "Experimentally Increasing
    Sedentary Behavior Results in Increased Anxiety in an Active Young
    Adult Population." *Journal of Affective Disorders* 204 (2016): 166–73;
    Meghan K. Edwards and Paul D. Loprinzi, "Effects of a Sedentary
    Behavior–Inducing Randomized Controlled Intervention on Depression
    and Mood Profile in Active Young Adults." *Mayo Clinic Proceedings* 91,
    no. 8 (2016): 984–98; Meghan K. Edwards and Paul D. Loprinzi,
    "Experimentally Increasing Sedentary Behavior Results in Decreased
    Life Satisfaction." *Health Promotion Perspectives* 7, no. 2 (2017): 88–94.

14 **The typical American takes 4,774 steps per day:** Tim Althoff et al.,
    "Large-Scale Physical Activity Data Reveal Worldwide Activity
    Inequality." *Nature* 547, no. 7663 (2017): 336–39.

15 For reviews of anatomical and physiological adaptations in humans that support running and hiking, see: Bramble and Lieberman, "Endurance Running and the Evolution of *Homo*"; Herman Pontzer, "Economy and Endurance in Human Evolution." *Current Biology* 27, no. 12 (2017): R613–21; Jay Schulkin, "Evolutionary Basis of Human Running and Its Impact on Neural Function." *Frontiers in Systems Neuroscience* 10 (2016): 59.

15 **As Herman Pontzer puts it:** Herman Pontzer, "The Exercise Paradox." *Scientific American,* February 2017. Quote appears on p. 27.

16 **high-intensity exercise causes an endorphin rush:** Tiina Saanijoki et al., "Opioid Release After High-Intensity Interval Training in Healthy Human Subjects." *Neuropsychopharmacology* 43, no. 2 (2018): 246–54; Henning Boecker et al., "The Runner's High: Opioidergic Mechanisms in the Human Brain." *Cerebral Cortex* 18, no. 11 (2008): 2523–31.

16 **descriptions of exercise-induced highs:** Patrick M. Whitehead, "The Runner's High Revisited: A Phenomenological Analysis." *Journal of Phenomenological Psychology* 47, no. 2 (2016): 183–98.

16–17 **Raichlen put regular runners through treadmill workouts:** David A. Raichlen et al., "Exercise-Induced Endocannabinoid Signaling Is Modulated by Intensity." *European Journal of Applied Physiology* 113, no. 4 (2013): 869–75.

17 **Raichlen decided to put pet dogs on his treadmill:** David A. Raichlen et al., "Wired to Run: Exercise-Induced Endocannabinoid Signaling in Humans and Cursorial Mammals with Implications for the 'Runner's High.'" *Journal of Experimental Biology* 215, no. 8 (2012): 1331–36.

17 **scientists have documented a similar increase in endocannabinoids:** Angelique G. Brellenthin et al., "Endocannabinoid and Mood Responses to Exercise in Adults with Varying Activity Levels." *Translational Journal of the American College of Sports Medicine* 2, no. 21 (2017): 138–45; E. Heyman et al., "Intense Exercise Increases Circulating Endocannabinoid and BDNF Levels in Humans—Possible Implications for Reward and Depression." *Psychoneuroendocrinology* 37, no. 6 (2012): 844–51; P. B. Sparling et al., "Exercise Activates the Endocannabinoid System." *NeuroReport* 14, no. 17 (2003): 2209–11; M. Feuerecker et al., "Effects of Exercise Stress on the Endocannabinoid System in Humans Under Field Conditions." *European Journal of Applied Physiology* 112, no. 7 (2012): 2777–81.

18 Quote and details about Julia are from a case study reported in Elizabeth Cassidy, Sandra Naylor, and Frances Reynolds, "The Meanings of Physiotherapy and Exercise for People Living with Progressive Cerebellar Ataxia: An Interpretative Phenomenological Analysis." *Disability and Rehabilitation* 40, no. 8 (2018): 894–904.

21–22 **As Foster told a reporter for ESPN:** David Fleming, "Slow and Steady Wins the Planet." *ESPN*, February 11, 2011; http://www.espn.com/espn /news/story?id=6110087.

23 **As runner Adharanand Finn observes:** Adharanand Finn, "Why We Love to Run." *The Guardian*, February 5, 2013; https://www .theguardian.com/lifeandstyle/the-running-blog/2013/feb/05/why-we -love-to-run.

23 **In clinical trials, the drug led to:** Robin Christensen et al., "Efficacy and Safety of the Weight-Loss Drug Rimonabant: A Meta-Analysis of Randomised Trials." *The Lancet* 370, no. 9600 (2007): P1706–13.

23 **As Morris describes the effects:** Hamilton Morris, "New Frontiers of Sobriety." *Vice*, July 31, 2009; https://www.vice.com/en_us/article /kwg8ny/new-frontiers-of-sobriety-984-v16n8.

24 **if you give the drug to rodents:** Brooke K. Keeney et al., "Differential Response to a Selective Cannabinoid Receptor Antagonist (SR141716: Rimonabant) in Female Mice from Lines Selectively Bred for High Voluntary Wheel-Running Behaviour." *Behavioural Pharmacology* 19, no. 8 (2008): 812–20; Sarah Dubreucq et al., "Ventral Tegmental Area Cannabinoid Type-1 Receptors Control Voluntary Exercise Performance." *Biological Psychiatry* 73, no. 9 (2013): 895–903.

24 **Blocking endocannabinoids also eliminates:** Johannes Fuss et al., "A Runner's High Depends on Cannabinoid Receptors in Mice." *Proceedings of the National Academy of Sciences of the USA* 112, no. 42 (2015): 13105–8.

25 **On days when people were active, stressful events:** Eli Puterman et al., "Physical Activity and Negative Affective Reactivity in Daily Life." *Health Psychology* 36, no. 12 (2017): 1186–94.

25 **In laboratory experiments, exercise:** Andreas Ströhle et al., "The Acute Antipanic and Anxiolytic Activity of Aerobic Exercise in Patients with Panic Disorder and Healthy Control Subjects." *Journal of Psychiatric Research* 43, no. 12 (2009): 1013–17.

26 **how the endocannabinoid system works:** Nora D. Volkow, Aidan J. Hampson, and Ruben D. Baler, "Don't Worry, Be Happy: Endocannabinoids and Cannabis at the Intersection of Stress and Reward." *Annual Review of Pharmacology and Toxicology* 57 (2017): 285–308.

26 **they are also about feeling close to others:** D. S. Karhson, A. Y. Hardan, and K. J. Parker, "Endocannabinoid Signaling in Social Functioning: an RDoC Perspective." *Translational Psychiatry* 6, no. 9 (2016): e905; Don Wei et al., "Endocannabinoid Signaling in the Control of Social Behavior." *Trends in Neurosciences* 40, no. 7 (2017): 385–96.

27 **Giving rats an endocannabinoid blocker:** Viviana Trezza, Petra J. J. Baarendse, and Louk J. M. J. Vanderschuren, "The Pleasures of Play:

Pharmacological Insights into Social Reward Mechanisms." *Trends in Pharmacological Sciences* 31, no. 10 (2010): 463–69.

27 **In mice, it makes new mothers:** Michal Schechter et al., "Blocking the Postpartum Mouse Dam's CB1 Receptors Impairs Maternal Behavior as Well as Offspring Development and Their Adult Social-Emotional Behavior." *Behavioural Brain Research* 226, no. 2 (2012): 481–92.

27 **"Over the course of a run":** I first heard John Cary's anecdote on Creating Our Own Lives podcast, then communicated via email. "My Best Conversations with Men Happen While Running." June 10, 2016; https://podtail.com/podcast/creating-our-own-lives/4-running-my -best-conversations-with-men-happ/.

27 **"My family will sometimes send me out running":** Alice Leadbeter, "Alice's Inspirational Running Story: Running Has Helped Me on So Many Levels." *261 Fearless*; http://www.261fearless.org/blog/l/alices -inspirational-running-story-running-has-helped-me-on-so-many -levels/.

27 **on days when people exercise:** Kevin C. Young et al., "The Cascade of Positive Events: Does Exercise on a Given Day Increase the Frequency of Additional Positive Events?" *Personality and Individual Differences* 120 (2018): 299–303.

27 **when spouses exercise together:** Jeremy B. Yorgason et al., "Marital Benefits of Daily Individual and Conjoint Exercise Among Older Couples." *Family Relations* 67, no. 2 (2018): 227–39.

28 **why humans have such big whites of the eyes:** Brian Hare, "Survival of the Friendliest: *Homo sapiens* Evolved via Selection for Prosociality." *Annual Review of Psychology* 68 (2017): 155–86.

28 **Another such adaptation is a neurobiological reward:** Jamil Zaki and Jason P. Mitchell, "Prosociality as a Form of Reward-Seeking." In Joshua David Greene, India Morrison, and Martin E. P. Seligman, eds., *Positive Neuroscience* (New York: Oxford University Press, 2016); Carolyn H. Declerck, Christophe Boone, and Griet Emonds, "When Do People Cooperate? The Neuroeconomics of Prosocial Decision Making." *Brain and Cognition* 81, no. 1 (2013): 95–117.

28 **Mutual cooperation activates brain regions:** James K. Rilling et al., "A Neural Basis for Social Cooperation." *Neuron* 35, no. 2 (2002): 395–405; Jean Decety et al., "The Neural Bases of Cooperation and Competition: An fMRI Investigation." *Neuroimage* 23, no. 2 (2004): 744–51.

29 **sitting around a fire encourages social bonding:** Christopher Dana Lynn, "Hearth and Campfire Influences on Arterial Blood Pressure: Defraying the Costs of the Social Brain Through Fireside Relaxation." *Evolutionary Psychology* 12, no. 5 (2014): 983–1003.

30 **An experiment at the Sapienza University of Rome:** Giovanni Di Bartolomeo and Stefano Papa, "The Effects of Physical Activity on

Social Interactions: The Case of Trust and Trustworthiness." *Journal of Sports Economics* (2017): doi.org/10.1177/1527002517717299.

31 **half the older adults in the UK:** Susan Davidson and Phil Rossall, "Evidence Review: Loneliness in Later Life." Age UK, July 2014. Available at: https://www.ageuk.org.uk/Documents/EN-GB/For -professionals/Research/Age%20UK%20Evidence%20Review%20on %20Loneliness%20July%202014.pdf.

31 **Two hundred thousand older adults in England and Wales:** Ceylan Yeginsu, "U.K. Appoints a Minister for Loneliness." *New York Times,* January 17, 2018; https://www.nytimes.com/2018/01/17/world/europe /uk-britain-loneliness.html.

31 **As one person who requested visits:** *Evaluation of GoodGym,* a 2015–2016 study conducted by Ecorys, funded by Nesta's Centre for Social Action Innovation Fund; https://media.nesta.org.uk/documents/good_gym _evaluation.pdf.

34 **ultra-distance runner Amit Sheth wrote:** Amit Sheth, *Dare to Run* (Mumbai: Sanjay and Company, 2011). Quote appears on p. 61.

34 **one of the ways that regular exercise changes your brain:** Valentina De Chiara et al., "Voluntary Exercise and Sucrose Consumption Enhance Cannabinoid CB1 Receptor Sensitivity in the Striatum." *Neuropsychopharmacology* 35, no. 2 (2010): 374–87; Matthew N. Hill et al., "Endogenous Cannabinoid Signaling Is Required for Voluntary Exercise-Induced Enhancement of Progenitor Cell Proliferation in the Hippocampus." *Hippocampus* 20, no. 4 (2010): 513–23.

Chapter 2: Getting Hooked

37 **As he later wrote:** Frederick Baekeland, "Exercise Deprivation: Sleep and Psychological Reactions." *Archives of General Psychiatry* 22, no. 4 (1970): 365–69.

37 **numerous studies have shown that for regular exercisers:** Julie A. Morgan et al., "Does Ceasing Exercise Induce Depressive Symptoms? A Systematic Review of Experimental Trials Including Immunological and Neurogenic Markers." *Journal of Affective Disorders* 234 (2018): 180–92; Eugene V. Aidman and Simon Woollard, "The Influence of Self-Reported Exercise Addiction on Acute Emotional and Physiological Responses to Brief Exercise Deprivation." *Psychology of Sport and Exercise* 4, no. 3 (2003): 225–36; Ali A. Weinstein, Christine Koehmstedt, and Willem J. Kop, "Mental Health Consequences of Exercise Withdrawal: A Systematic Review." *General Hospital Psychiatry* 49 (2017): 11–18.

38 **exercise scientist Attila Szabo declared:** Attila Szabo, "Studying the Psychological Impact of Exercise Deprivation: Are Experimental Studies Hopeless?" *Journal of Sport Behavior* 21, no. 2 (1998): 139–47.

38 **This phenomenon—known as** *attention capture*: Boris Cheval et al., "Behavioral and Neural Evidence of the Rewarding Value of Exercise Behaviors: A Systematic Review." *Sports Medicine* 48, no. 6 (2018): 1389–1404.

38 **when self-proclaimed exercise addicts view images:** Yu Jin Kim et al., "The Neural Mechanism of Exercise Addiction as Determined by Functional Magnetic Resonance Imaging (fMRI)." *Journal of Korean Association of Physical Education and Sport for Girls and Women* 32, no. 1 (2018): 69–80.

38 **A small percentage of exercisers also show symptoms:** Kata Mónok et al., "Psychometric Properties and Concurrent Validity of Two Exercise Addiction Measures: A Population Wide Study." *Psychology of Sport and Exercise* 13, no. 6 (2012): 739–46.

38 **One forty-six-year-old long-distance runner:** Joshua Justin Cook, "The Relationship Between Mental Health and Ultra-Running: A Case Study," 2018. *Theses and Dissertations.* 2850 http://scholarworks.uark .edu/etd/2850.

39 **Theodore Garland Jr. told a** *New Yorker* **journalist:** Nicola Twilley, "A Pill to Make Exercise Obsolete." *The New Yorker,* November 6, 2017, 30–35.

40 **Exercise physiologist Samuele Marcora has proposed:** Samuele Marcora, "Can Doping Be a Good Thing? Using Psychoactive Drugs to Facilitate Physical Activity Behaviour." *Sports Medicine* 46, no. 1 (2016): 1–5.

41 **Chronic use of such a drug eventually flips:** Eric J. Nestler, "ΔFosB: A Molecular Switch for Reward." *Journal of Drug and Alcohol Research* 2 (2013): article ID 235651.

41 **These proteins trigger long-lasting changes:** Nora D. Volkow and Marisela Morales, "The Brain on Drugs: From Reward to Addiction." *Cell* 162, no. 4 (2015): 712–25.

41 **Scientists have observed these changes:** Deanna L. Wallace et al., "The Influence of ΔFosB in the Nucleus Accumbens on Natural Reward-Related Behavior." *Journal of Neuroscience* 28, no. 41 (2008): 10272–77.

41 **running also flips the molecular switch:** Martin Werme et al., "ΔFosB Regulates Wheel Running." *Journal of Neuroscience* 22, no. 18 (2002): 8133–38.

41 **In laboratory studies with rats:** Martin Werme et al., "Running and Cocaine Both Upregulate Dynorphin mRNA in Medial Caudate Putamen." *European Journal of Neuroscience* 12, no. 8 (2000): 2967–74.

42 **they go on running binges:** Anthony Ferreira et al., "Spontaneous Appetence for Wheel-Running: A Model of Dependency on Physical Activity in Rat." *European Psychiatry* 21, no. 8 (2006): 580–88.

42 **Two weeks of wheel-running is insufficient:** Benjamin N. Greenwood et al., "Long-Term Voluntary Wheel Running Is Rewarding and

Produces Plasticity in the Mesolimbic Reward Pathway." *Behavioural Brain Research* 217, no. 2 (2011): 354–62.

42 **sedentary adults who begin high-intensity training:** Jennifer J. Heisz et al., "Enjoyment for High-Intensity Interval Exercise Increases During the First Six Weeks of Training: Implications for Promoting Exercise Adherence in Sedentary Adults." *PLOS ONE* 11, no. 12 (2016): e0168534.

42 **One study of new members at a gym:** Navin Kaushal and Ryan E. Rhodes, "Exercise Habit Formation in New Gym Members: A Longitudinal Study." *Journal of Behavioral Medicine* 38, no. 4 (2015): 652–63.

43 **such as the young single mother:** Barbara Walsh et al., "'Net Mums': A Narrative Account of Participants' Experiences Within a Netball Intervention." *Qualitative Research in Sport, Exercise and Health* 10, no. 5 (2018): 604–19.

43 **"I know I'm in freedom when I move":** Quote appears as part of a case study in Rebecca Y. Concepcion and Vicki Ebbeck, "Examining the Physical Activity Experiences of Survivors of Domestic Violence in Relation to Self-Views." *Journal of Sport and Exercise Psychology* 27, no. 2 (2005): 197–211.

47 **In 1976, marathon runner Ian Thompson:** Valerie Andrews, "The Joy of Jogging," *New York* 10, no. 1 (1976): 61. Accessed via: https://books .google.com/books?id=mYQpAQAAIAAJ.

47 **the conditioned rush that scientists call the *pleasure gloss*:** J. Wayne Aldridge and Kent C. Berridge, "Neural Coding of Pleasure: Rose-Tinted Glasses of the Ventral Pallidum." In M. L. Kringelbach and K. C. Berridge, eds., *Pleasures of the Brain* (New York: Oxford University Press, 2010), 62–73.

47 **Psychiatrist Benjamin Kissin noted:** Benjamin Kissin, "The Disease Concept of Alcoholism." In R. G. Smart et al., *Research Advances in Alcohol and Drug Problems* (New York: Plenum Press, 1983), 93–126. Example cited on 113.

52 **Chronic drug use also lowers:** Nora D. Volkow, George F. Koob, and A. Thomas McLellan, "Neurobiologic Advances from the Brain Disease Model of Addiction." *New England Journal of Medicine* 374, no. 4 (2016): 363–71.

52 **the dark side of addiction:** George F. Koob and Michel Le Moal, "Plasticity of Reward Neurocircuitry and the 'Dark Side' of Drug Addiction." *Nature Neuroscience* 8, no. 11 (2005): 1442–44; George F. Koob and Michel Le Moal, "Addiction and the Brain Antireward System." *Annual Review of Psychology* 59 (2008): 29–53.

52 **exercise leads to higher circulating levels:** Christopher M. Olsen, "Natural Rewards, Neuroplasticity, and Non-Drug Addictions." *Neuropharmacology* 61, no. 7 (2011): 1109–22; Lisa S. Robison et al.,

"Exercise Reduces Dopamine D1R and Increases D2R in Rats: Implications for Addiction." *Medicine and Science in Sports and Exercise* 50, no. 8 (2018): 1596–1602.

52 **In both animal and human studies:** For some examples, see Maciej S. Buchowski et al., "Aerobic Exercise Training Reduces Cannabis Craving and Use in Non-Treatment Seeking Cannabis-Dependent Adults." *PLOS ONE* 6, no. 3 (2011): e17465; Dongshi Wang et al., "Aerobic Exercise Training Ameliorates Craving and Inhibitory Control in Methamphetamine Dependencies: A Randomized Controlled Trial and Event-Related Potential Study." *Psychology of Sport and Exercise* 30 (2017): 82–90; Maryam Alizadeh, Mahdi Zahedi-Khorasani, and Hossein Miladi-Gorji, "Treadmill Exercise Attenuates the Severity of Physical Dependence, Anxiety, Depressive-Like Behavior and Voluntary Morphine Consumption in Morphine Withdrawn Rats Receiving Methadone Maintenance Treatment." *Neuroscience Letters* 681 (2018): 73–77; Dongshi Wang et al., "Impact of Physical Exercise on Substance Use Disorders: A Meta-Analysis." *PLOS ONE* 9, no. 10 (2014): e110728.

52 **adults in treatment for methamphetamine abuse:** Chelsea L. Robertson et al., "Effect of Exercise Training on Striatal Dopamine D2/D3 Receptors in Methamphetamine Users During Behavioral Treatment." *Neuropsychopharmacology* 41, no. 6 (2016): 1629–36.

53 **Over time, deep brain stimulation:** Thomas E. Schlaepfer et al., "Rapid Effects of Deep Brain Stimulation for Treatment-Resistant Major Depression." *Biological Psychiatry* 73, no. 12 (2013): 1204–12; Manoj P. Dandekar et al., "Increased Dopamine Receptor Expression and Anti-Depressant Response Following Deep Brain Stimulation of the Medial Forebrain Bundle." *Journal of Affective Disorders* 217 (2017): 80–88.

53 **A meta-analysis of twenty-five randomized clinical trials:** Felipe B. Schuch et al., "Exercise as a Treatment for Depression: A Meta-Analysis Adjusting for Publication Bias." *Journal of Psychiatric Research* 77 (2016): 42–51.

53 **Another review of thirteen studies:** Gioia Mura et al., "Exercise as an Add-On Strategy for the Treatment of Major Depressive Disorder: A Systematic Review." *CNS Spectrums* 19, no. 6 (2014): 496–508.

53 **This loss leads to less enjoyment:** Linh C. Dang et al., "Reduced Effects of Age on Dopamine D2 Receptor Levels in Physically Active Adults." *NeuroImage* 148 (2017): 123–29.

54 **a selective breeding experiment with mice:** Justin S. Rhodes and Petra Majdak, "Physical Activity and Reward: The Role of Dopamine." In Panteleimon Ekkekakis, ed., *Routledge Handbook of Physical Activity and Mental Health* (New York: Routledge, 2013).

55 **as the human species evolved, we developed a shared genome:** Ayland C. Letsinger et al., "Alleles Associated with Physical Activity Levels Are Estimated to Be Older Than Anatomically Modern Humans." *PloS ONE* 14, no. 4 (2019): e0216155.

55 **Maybe everything we know about how movement affects the human brain:** For an interesting discussion of how our ancestors' need to be active led to the modern neuroprotective benefits of exercise, see David A. Raichlen and Gene E. Alexander, "Adaptive Capacity: An Evolutionary Neuroscience Model Linking Exercise, Cognition, and Brain Health." *Trends in Neurosciences* 40, no. 7 (2017): 408–21.

55 **50 percent of the variability in physical activity:** Xueying Zhang and John R. Speakman, "Genetic Factors Associated with Human Physical Activity: Are Your Genes Too Tight to Prevent You Exercising?" *Endocrinology* (2019): https://doi.org/10.1210/en.2018-00873; J. Timothy Lightfoot et al., "Biological/Genetic Regulation of Physical Activity Level: Consensus from GenBioPAC." *Medicine & Science in Sports & Exercise* 50, no. 4 (2018): 863–73.

55–56 **heritability estimates drop:** Nienke M. Schutte et al., "Heritability of the Affective Response to Exercise and Its Correlation to Exercise Behavior." *Psychology of Sport and Exercise* 31 (2017): 139–48.

58 **recent large-scale genome-wide association studies:** For examples, see Yann C. Klimentidis et al., "Genome-Wide Association Study of Habitual Physical Activity in Over 377,000 UK Biobank Participants Identifies Multiple Variants Including CADM2 and APOE." *International Journal of Obesity* 42 (2018): 1161–76; Xiaochen Lin et al., "Genetic Determinants for Leisure-Time Physical Activity." *Medicine and Science in Sports and Exercise* 50, no. 8 (2018): 1620–28; Aiden Doherty et al., "GWAS Identifies 14 Loci for Device-Measured Physical Activity and Sleep Duration." *Nature communications* 9, no. 1 (2018): 5257.

59 **Scientists have identified several strands of DNA, on multiple genes:** For examples, see Marcus K. Taylor et al., "A Genetic Risk Factor for Major Depression and Suicidal Ideation Is Mitigated by Physical Activity." *Psychiatry Research* 249 (2017): 304–6; Helmuth Haslacher et al., "Physical Exercise Counteracts Genetic Susceptibility to Depression." *Neuropsychobiology* 71, no. 3 (2015): 168–75; Dharani Keyan and Richard A. Bryant, "Acute Exercise-Induced Enhancement of Fear Inhibition Is Moderated by BDNF Val66Met Polymorphism." *Translational Psychiatry* 9, no. 1 (2019): 131.

60 **physical activity immediately decreases anxiety:** Matthew P. Herring, Mats Hallgren, and Mark J. Campbell, "Acute Exercise Effects on Worry, State Anxiety, and Feelings of Energy and Fatigue Among Young Women with Probable Generalized Anxiety Disorder: A Pilot Study." *Psychology of Sport and Exercise* 33 (2017): 31–36; Matthew P. Herring et al.,

"Acute Exercise Effects Among Young Adults with Subclinical Generalized Anxiety Disorder: Replication and Expansion." *Medicine & Science in Sports & Exercise* 50, no. 5S (2018): 249–50; Serge Brand et al., "Acute Bouts of Exercising Improved Mood, Rumination and Social Interaction in Inpatients with Mental Disorders." *Frontiers in Psychology* 9 (2018): 249.

60 **this effect becomes even more pronounced:** K. M. Lucibello, J. Parker, and J. J. Heisz, "Examining a Training Effect on the State Anxiety Response to an Acute Bout of Exercise in Low and High Anxious Individuals." *Journal of Affective Disorders* 247 (2019): 29–35.

60 **A 2017 meta-analysis of exercise interventions:** Brendon Stubbs et al., "An Examination of the Anxiolytic Effects of Exercise for People with Anxiety and Stress-Related Disorders: A Meta-Analysis." *Psychiatry Research* 249 (2017): 102–8.

62 **it also targets regions of the brain that regulate anxiety:** Julie A. Morgan, Frances Corrigan, and Bernhard T. Baune, "Effects of Physical Exercise on Central Nervous System Functions: A Review of Brain Region Specific Adaptations." *Journal of Molecular Psychiatry* 3, no. 1 (2015): 3.

62 **In laboratory studies with rats:** N. R. Sciolino et al., "Galanin Mediates Features of Neural and Behavioral Stress Resilience Afforded by Exercise." *Neuropharmacology* 89 (2015): 255–64.

62 **In humans, exercising three times a week:** Karl-Jürgen Bär et al., "Hippocampal-Brainstem Connectivity Associated with Vagal Modulation After an Intense Exercise Intervention in Healthy Men." *Frontiers in Neuroscience* 10 (2016): 145.

62 **research even suggests that lactate:** Nabil Karnib et al., "Lactate Is an Antidepressant That Mediates Resilience to Stress by Modulating the Hippocampal Levels and Activity of Histone Deacetylases." *Neuropsychopharmacology* (2019): 10.1038/s41386-019-0313-z; Patrizia Proia et al., "Lactate as a Metabolite and a Regulator in the Central Nervous System." *International Journal of Molecular Sciences* 17, no. 9 (2016): 1450.

62–63 **In a laboratory experiment at the University of Wisconsin:** Justin S. Rhodes, Theodore Garland Jr., and Stephen C. Gammie, "Patterns of Brain Activity Associated with Variation in Voluntary Wheel-Running Behavior." *Behavioral Neuroscience* 117, no. 6 (2003): 1243–56.

63 **When heartbroken young adults:** Helen E. Fisher et al., "Reward, Addiction, and Emotion Regulation Systems Associated with Rejection in Love." *Journal of Neurophysiology* 104, no. 1 (2010): 51–60.

63 **When a mother gazes at her baby:** Shir Atzil et al., "Dopamine in the Medial Amygdala Network Mediates Human Bonding." *Proceedings of the National Academy of Sciences of the USA* 114, no. 9 (2017): 2361–66.

63 **The scent of her infant's skin:** Johan N. Lundström et al., "Maternal Status Regulates Cortical Responses to the Body Odor of Newborns." *Frontiers in Psychology* 4 (2013): 597.

63 **One of my favorite headlines:** Sophie Haslett, "'I could just eat you up!' The scientific reason behind a mother's desire to nuzzle, nibble or EVEN gobble her baby revealed . . . and don't worry—it's perfectly natural." *Daily Mail Australia,* April 6, 2016. http://www.dailymail.co.uk/femail/article -3525665/Why-science-says-mother-s-wish-eat-baby-entirely-natural.html.

64 **One research paper described missing:** James P. Burkett and Larry J. Young, "The Behavioral, Anatomical and Pharmacological Parallels Between Social Attachment, Love and Addiction." *Psychopharmacology* 224, no. 1 (2012): 1–26.

64 **The same brain responses that scientists compare:** Bianca P. Acevedo, "Neural Correlates of Human Attachment: Evidence from fMRI Studies of Adult Pair-Bonding." In Vivian Zayas and Cindy Hazan, eds., *Bases of Adult Attachment* (New York: Springer, 2015), 185–94.

64 **The burst of dopamine in a mother's brain:** Atzil et al., "Dopamine in the Medial Amygdala Network Mediates Human Bonding."

64 **In long-term happily married couples:** Bianca P. Acevedo et al., "Neural Correlates of Long-Term Intense Romantic Love." *Social Cognitive and Affective Neuroscience* 7, no. 2 (2012): 145–59.

64 **And when a widow or widower:** Mary-Frances O'Connor et al., "Craving Love? Enduring Grief Activates Brain's Reward Center." *Neuroimage* 42, no. 2 (2008): 969–72.

65 **the more the parents describe their babies:** Pilyoung Kim et al., "The Plasticity of Human Maternal Brain: Longitudinal Changes in Brain Anatomy During the Early Postpartum Period." *Behavioral Neuroscience* 124, no. 5 (2010): 695; Pilyoung Kim et al., "Neural Plasticity in Fathers of Human Infants." *Social Neuroscience* 9, no. 5 (2014): 522–35.

Chapter 3: Collective Joy

68 **Durkheim coined the term** *collective effervescence*: Émile Durkheim, *The Elementary Forms of the Religious Life* (1912), English translation by Joseph Ward Swain, 1915 (New York: The Free Press, 1965).

70 **what modern researchers refer to as** *collective joy*: The term *collective joy* was proposed by Barbara Ehrenreich in Barbara Ehrenreich, *Dancing in the Streets: A History of Collective Joy* (New York: Henry Holt, 2007). See also Edith Turner, *Communitas: The Anthropology of Collective Joy* (New York: Palgrave Macmillan, 2012).

70–71 **"As the dancer loses himself in the dance":** A. R. Radcliffe-Brown, *The Andaman Islanders* (1st British ed., 1922; New York: Cambridge University Press, 1933). Quote appears on p. 252. Accessed at https://archive.org /details/TheAndamanIslandersAStudyInSocialAnthropology.

71 **Tarr ran an experiment:** Bronwyn Tarr et al., "Synchrony and Exertion During Dance Independently Raise Pain Threshold and Encourage Social Bonding." *Biology Letters* 11, no. 10 (2015): doi: 10.1098/rsbl.2015.076720150767.

71 **in a series of silent discos:** Bronwyn Tarr, Jacques Launay, and Robin I. M. Dunbar, "Silent Disco: Dancing in Synchrony Leads to Elevated Pain Thresholds and Social Closeness." *Evolution and Human Behavior* 37, no. 5 (2016): 343–49.

72 **collective joy is driven in part by endorphins:** Bronwyn Tarr et al., "Naltrexone Blocks Endorphins Released When Dancing in Synchrony." *Adaptive Human Behavior and Physiology* 3, no. 3 (2017): 241–54.

72 **strangers who practiced yoga together:** Ronald Fischer et al., "How Do Rituals Affect Cooperation? An Experimental Field Study Comparing Nine Ritual Types." *Human Nature* 24, no. 2 (2013): 115–25.

74–75 **your brain interprets the other bodies:** Stephanie Cacioppo et al., "You Are in Sync with Me: Neural Correlates of Interpersonal Synchrony with a Partner." *Neuroscience* 277 (2014): 842–58.

75 **the *kinaesthetics of togetherness*:** Tommi Himberg et al., "Coordinated Interpersonal Behaviour in Collective Dance Improvisation: The Aesthetics of Kinaesthetic Togetherness." *Behavioral Sciences (Basel)* 8, no. 2 (2018): 23.

75 **that individual's sense of personal space transfers:** I learned this fascinating fact from Anil Ananthaswamy, *The Man Who Wasn't There: Tales from the Edge of the Self* (New York: Penguin, 2016).

77 **In March 2016, CrossFit gym owner Brandon Bergeron:** Emily Lavin, "Community Effort Helps Grass Valley CrossFit Find New Home." *The Union,* July 14, 2016; https://www.theunion.com/news/business/community-effort-helps-grass-valley-crossfit-find-new-home/.

77 **synchronized movement . . . encourages us to share and help:** Miriam Rennung and Anja S. Göritz, "Prosocial Consequences of Interpersonal Synchrony: A Meta-Analysis." *Zeitschrift für Psychologie* 224, no. 3 (2016): 168–89; Reneeta Mogan, Ronald Fischer, and Joseph A. Bulbulia, "To Be in Synchrony or Not? A Meta-Analysis of Synchrony's Effects on Behavior, Perception, Cognition and Affect." *Journal of Experimental Social Psychology* 72 (2017): 13–20; Paul Reddish et al., "Collective Synchrony Increases Prosociality Towards Non-Performers and Outgroup Members." *British Journal of Social Psychology* 55, no. 4 (2016): 722–38.

77 **Even babies show this effect:** Laura K. Cirelli, "How Interpersonal Synchrony Facilitates Early Prosocial Behavior." *Current Opinion in Psychology* 20 (2018): 35–39.

78 **We humans have our own forms of social grooming:** Robin I. M. Dunbar, "The Anatomy of Friendship." *Trends in Cognitive Sciences* 22, no. 1 (2018): 32–51.

78 **group forms of social grooming make it possible:** Cole Robertson et al., "Rapid Partner Switching May Facilitate Increased Broadcast Group Size in Dance Compared with Conversation Groups." *Ethology* 123, no. 10 (2017): 736–47.

78 **Across cultures, most people's social networks:** Dunbar, "The Anatomy of Friendship."

79 **fellows at Harvard Divinity School, observed CrossFit communities:** Mark Oppenheimer, "When Some Turn to Church, Others Go to CrossFit." *New York Times*, November 27, 2015; Angie Thurston on "Boutique Fitness Craze," *On Point* radio broadcast, January 6, 2016; http://www.wbur.org/onpoint/2016/01/07/soulcycle-devotion-explanation.

81 **the Jogging over a Distance app:** Florian "Floyd" Mueller et al., "Jogging over a Distance: The Influence of Design in Parallel Exertion Games." In *Proceedings of the 5th ACM SIGGRAPH Symposium on Video Games*, Los Angeles, CA, July 25–29, 2010, 63–68.

82 **the world's first robotic jogging companion:** Florian "Floyd" Mueller et al., "13 Game Lenses for Designing Diverse Interactive Jogging Systems." In *Proceedings of the Annual Symposium on Computer-Human Interaction in Play*, ACM, 2017, 43–56.

83 **Tarr has recently replicated her dance experiments in virtual reality:** Bronwyn Tarr, Mel Slater, and Emma Cohen, "Synchrony and Social Connection in Immersive Virtual Reality." *Scientific Reports* 8, no. 1 (2018): 3693.

85 **When William H. McNeill was drafted:** William H. McNeill, *Keeping Together in Time: Dance and Drill in Human History* (Cambridge, MA: Harvard University Press, 1995). Quotes from pp. 1–2. Additional details about his basic training are from William McNeill, *The Pursuit of Truth: A Historian's Memoir* (Lexington: University Press of Kentucky, 2005), 45–46.

85 **Psychologists call this sense of empowerment:** Elisabeth Pacherie, "The Phenomenology of Joint Action: Self-Agency Versus Joint Agency." In Axel Seemann, ed., *Joint Attention: New Developments in Psychology, Philosophy of Mind, and Social Neuroscience* (Cambridge, MA: MIT Press, 2012), 343–89.

85 **The Aztecs, Spartans, and Zulus all used:** William H. McNeill, *The Pursuit of Power: Technology, Armed Force, and Society since A.D. 1000* (Chicago: University of Chicago Press, 1982).

86 **humans might have developed synchronized movement as a defense:** Joachim Richter and Roya Ostovar, "'It Don't Mean a Thing if

It Ain't Got That Swing'—an Alternative Concept for Understanding the Evolution of Dance and Music in Human Beings." *Frontiers in Human Neuroscience* 10 (2016): 485.

86 **Many species deploy strategies:** Charlotte Duranton and Florence Gaunet, "Behavioural Synchronization from an Ethological Perspective: Overview of Its Adaptive Value." *Adaptive Behavior* 24, no. 3 (2016): 181–91; Valeria Senigaglia et al., "The Role of Synchronized Swimming as Affiliative and Anti-Predatory Behavior in Long-Finned Pilot Whales." *Behavioural Processes* 91, no. 1 (2012): 8–14.

86–87 **When participants heard synchronized steps:** Daniel M. T. Fessler and Colin Holbrook, "Synchronized Behavior Increases Assessments of the Formidability and Cohesion of Coalitions." *Evolution and Human Behavior* 37, no. 6 (2016): 502–9.

87 **Any group moving in unison is seen by others:** Daniël Lakens and Mariëlle Stel, "If They Move in Sync, They Must Feel in Sync: Movement Synchrony Leads to Attributions of Rapport and Entitativity." *Social Cognition* 29, no. 1 (2011): 1–14.

87 **When people move together:** Daniel M. T. Fessler and Colin Holbrook. "Marching into Battle: Synchronized Walking Diminishes the Conceptualized Formidability of an Antagonist in Men." *Biology Letters* 10, no. 8 (2014): doi: 10.1098/rsbl.2014.0592.

87 **Studies of real-world marches and demonstrations:** Dario Páez et al., "Psychosocial Effects of Perceived Emotional Synchrony in Collective Gatherings." *Journal of Personality and Social Psychology* 108, no. 5 (2015): 711–29.

89 **the effects of participating in charity athletic events:** Kevin Filo and Alexandra Coghlan, "Exploring the Positive Psychology Domains of Well-Being Activated Through Charity Sport Event Experiences." *Event Management* 20, no. 2 (2016): 181–99.

91 **Those who increased their participation in group exercise:** Taishi Tsuji et al., "Reducing Depressive Symptoms After the Great East Japan Earthquake in Older Survivors Through Group Exercise Participation and Regular Walking: A Prospective Observational Study." *BMJ Open* 7, no. 3 (2017): e013706.

92 **Jacob Devaney, who rebuilt homes in New Orleans:** Jacob Devaney, "Research Shows Dancing Makes You Feel Better." *Uplift*, December 14, 2015.

92–93 **Groups will often synchronize:** Erwan Codrons et al., "Spontaneous Group Synchronization of Movements and Respiratory Rhythms." *PLOS ONE* 9, no. 9 (2014): e107538.

93 **Cognitive scientist Mark Changizi uses the word *nature-harnessing*:** Mark Changizi, *Harnessed: How Language and Music Mimicked Nature and Transformed Ape to Man* (Dallas: BenBella Books, 2011). Quote is on p. 5.

93–94 **the more you get your heart rate up:** Joshua Conrad Jackson et al., "Synchrony and Physiological Arousal Increase Cohesion and Cooperation in Large Naturalistic Groups." *Scientific Reports* 8, no. 1 (2018): 127.

94 **Adding music has the same enhancing effect:** Jan Stupacher et al., "Music Strengthens Prosocial Effects of Interpersonal Synchronization—If You Move in Time with the Beat." *Journal of Experimental Social Psychology* 72 (2017): 39–44.

94 **happy sweat has a different odor:** Jasper H. B. de Groot et al., "A Sniff of Happiness." *Psychological Science* 26, no. 6 (2015): 684–700.

94 **The scent of joy . . . appears to be culturally universal:** Jasper H. B. de Groot et al., "Beyond the West: Chemosignaling of Emotions Transcends Ethno-Cultural Boundaries." *Psychoneuroendocrinology* 98 (2018): 177–85.

94 **Analyzing the dance rituals of the Andaman Islanders:** Radcliffe-Brown, *The Andaman Islanders.* Quote appears on p. 248.

95 **people who have a prosocial orientation:** Joanne Lumsden et al., "Who Syncs? Social Motives and Interpersonal Coordination." *Journal of Experimental Social Psychology* 48, no. 3 (2012): 746–51.

95 **"Euphoric response to keeping together":** McNeill, *Keeping Together in Time: Dance and Drill in Human History.* Quote appears on p. 150.

Chapter 4: Let Yourself Be Moved

97–98 **Musicologists call this urge** *groove:* Petr Janata, Stefan T. Tomic, and Jason M. Haberman, "Sensorimotor Coupling in Music and the Psychology of the Groove." *Journal of Experimental Psychology: General* 141, no. 1 (2012): 54–75.

98 **Newborns . . . can detect a regular beat:** István Winkler et al., "Newborn Infants Detect the Beat in Music." *Proceedings of the National Academy of Sciences of the USA* 106, no. 7 (2009): 2468–71.

98 **Infants rock their feet:** Marcel Zentner and Tuomas Eerola, "Rhythmic Engagement with Music in Infancy." *Proceedings of the National Academy of Sciences of the USA* 107, no. 13 (2010): 5768–73; Beatriz Ilari, "Rhythmic Engagement with Music in Early Childhood: A Replication and Extension." *Journal of Research in Music Education* 62 (2015): 332–43.

98 **Music activates the so-called motor loop:** Chelsea L. Gordon, Patrice R. Cobb, and Ramesh Balasubramaniam, "Recruitment of the Motor System During Music Listening: An ALE Meta-Analysis of fMRI Data." *PLOS ONE* 13, no. 11 (2018): e0207213.

98 **The stronger the musical beat:** Katja Kornysheva et al., "Tuning-in to the Beat: Aesthetic Appreciation of Musical Rhythms Correlates with a Premotor Activity Boost." *Human Brain Mapping* 31, no. 1 (2010): 48–64.

98 **"When listening to music, we listen with our muscles":** Oliver Sacks, *A Leg to Stand On* (New York: Simon & Schuster/Touchstone, 1998). Quote appears on p. 13. Sacks claims to be quoting Nietzsche, although I could not find any original source confirming this quote.

99 **"Every weary and footsore soldier":** Robert Goldthwaite Carter, *Four Brothers in Blue, or Sunshine and Shadow of the War of the Rebellion: A Story of the Great Civil War from Bull Run to Appomattox* (Washington, DC: Press of Gibson Bros., Inc., 1913). Quote appears on p. 297. Accessed at https://archive.org/details/cu31924032780623.

99 **Seventy-six-year-old Tucker Andersen:** Juliet Macur, "A Marathon Without Music? Runners with Headphones Balk at Policy." *New York Times,* November 1, 2007.

100 **The brain responds to music it enjoys:** Anne J. Blood and Robert J. Zatorre, "Intensely Pleasurable Responses to Music Correlate with Activity in Brain Regions Implicated in Reward and Emotion." *Proceedings of the National Academy of Sciences of the USA* 98, no. 20 (2001): 11818–23; Valorie N. Salimpoor et al., "Anatomically Distinct Dopamine Release During Anticipation and Experience of Peak Emotion to Music." *Nature Neuroscience* 14, no. 2 (2011): 257–62.

100 **musicologists describe music as *ergogenic*:** Marc Leman, *The Expressive Moment: How Interaction (with Music) Shapes Human Empowerment* (Cambridge, MA: MIT Press, 2016).

100 **middle-aged patients with diabetes:** Karan Sarode et al., "Does Music Impact Exercise Capacity During Cardiac Stress Test? A Single Blinded Pilot Randomized Controlled Study." *Journal of the American College of Cardiology* 71, no. 11 (2018): A400.

101 **adding a soundtrack helps rowers, sprinters, and swimmers:** Mária Rendi, Attila Szabo, and Tamás Szabó, "Performance Enhancement with Music in Rowing Sprint." *The Sport Psychologist* 22, no. 2 (2008): 175–82. Stuart D. Simpson and Costas I. Karageorghis, "The Effects of Synchronous Music on 400-Metre Sprint Performance." *Journal of Sports Sciences* 24, no. 10 (2006): 1095–102; Costas Karageorghis et al., "Psychological, Psychophysical, and Ergogenic Effects of Music in Swimming." *Psychology of Sport and Exercise* 14, no. 4 (2013): 560–68.

101 **Runners can tolerate extreme heat:** Luke Nikol et al., "The Heat Is On: Effects of Synchronous Music on Psychophysiological Parameters and Running Performance in Hot and Humid Conditions." *Frontiers in Psychology* 9 (2018): 1114.

101 **triathletes can push themselves farther:** Peter C. Terry et al., "Effects of Synchronous Music on Treadmill Running Among Elite Triathletes." *Journal of Science and Medicine in Sport* 15, no. 1 (2012): 52–57.

101 **music is a legal performance-enhancing drug:** Edith Van Dyck and Marc Leman, "Ergogenic Effect of Music During Running

Performance." *Annals of Sports Medicine and Research* 3, no. 6 (2016): 1082.

104 **listening to "Eye of the Tiger":** Marcelo Bigliassi et al., "Cerebral Mechanisms Underlying the Effects of Music During a Fatiguing Isometric Ankle-Dorsiflexion Task." *Psychophysiology* 53, no. 10 (2016): 1472–83.

105 **it colors your interpretation:** Jonathan M. Bird et al., "Effects of Music and Music-Video on Core Affect During Exercise at the Lactate Threshold." *Psychology of Music* 44, no. 6 (2016): 1471–87.

105 **researchers asked women to say out loud:** Elaine A. Rose and Gaynor Parfitt, "Pleasant for Some and Unpleasant for Others: A Protocol Analysis of the Cognitive Factors That Influence Affective Responses to Exercise." *International Journal of Behavioral Nutrition and Physical Activity* 7 (2010): 1–15.

111 **psychologists and musicologists at Dartmouth College:** Beau Sievers et al., "Music and Movement Share a Dynamic Structure That Supports Universal Expressions of Emotion." *Proceedings of the National Academy of Sciences of the USA* 110, no. 1 (2013): 70–75.

112 **Different movements reliably produced distinct emotions:** Tal Shafir et al., "Emotion Regulation Through Execution, Observation, and Imagery of Emotional Movements." *Brain and Cognition* 82, no. 2 (2013): 219–27; Tal Shafir, Rachelle P. Tsachor, and Kathleen B. Welch, "Emotion Regulation Through Movement: Unique Sets of Movement Characteristics Are Associated With and Enhance Basic Emotions." *Frontiers in Psychology* 6 (2016): 02030.

113 **"The individual shouts and jumps for joy":** Radcliffe-Brown, *The Andaman Islanders.* Quote appears on p. 247.

113 **the jumping dance of the Maasai warriors in Kenya:** Watch the dance at https://www.youtube.com/watch?v=ZA4bAuAoEsU.

113 **I met Miriam:** "Miriam" is a pseudonym used at the request of the individual. No other details or quotes have been altered in this story.

116–17 **The mask is often misread:** Rachel Schwartz and Marc D. Pell, "When Emotion and Expression Diverge: The Social Costs of Parkinson's Disease." *Journal of Clinical and Experimental Neuropsychology* 39, no. 3 (2017): 211–30.

117 **Music triggers spontaneous facial expressions:** Lars-Olov Lundqvist et al., "Emotional Responses to Music: Experience, Expression, and Physiology." *Psychology of Music* 37, no. 1 (2009): 61–90.

117 **dance classes modeled on the Dance for PD program:** Lisa Heiberger et al., "Impact of a Weekly Dance Class on the Functional Mobility and on the Quality of Life of Individuals with Parkinson's Disease." *Frontiers in Aging Neuroscience* 3 (2011): 14.

121 **neurologist Oliver Sacks told the story:** "Forever Young: Music and Aging." Hearing before the Special Committee on Aging, United States Senate. Washington, D.C., August 1, 1991. Hearing 102-545. Testimony transcript available at: https://www.aging.senate.gov/imo/media/doc/publications/811991.pdf

121 **"It stirs some barbaric instinct":** Virginia Woolf, "A Dance at Queen's Gate." In *A Passionate Apprentice: The Early Journals, 1897–1909*, Mitchell A. Leaska, ed. (San Diego: Harcourt Brace Jovanovich, 1990).

122 **"Even when I'm just listening":** Jennifer J. Nicol, "Body, Time, Space and Relationship in the Music Listening Experiences of Women with Chronic Illness." *Psychology of Music* 38, no. 3 (2010): 351–67.

Chapter 5: Overcoming Obstacles

127 **"I wanted to see how strong I could become":** Araliya Ming Senerat's quote comes from an Instagram post. Her story is included with permission. For more stories about the psychological benefits of powerlifting among women, see: https://www.buzzfeed.com/sallytamarkin/badass-people-who-lift-weights-to-heal-fight-oppression.

127 **Widdicombe likened it to a rite of passage:** Lizzie Widdicombe, "In Cold Mud." *The New Yorker*, January 27, 2014.

128 **he was routinely shocked by cattle fences:** Anecdote appears in Will Dean, *It Takes a Tribe: Building the Tough Mudder Movement* (New York: Penguin, 2017), 114–15.

131 **But sometimes shocking rats doesn't make them helpless:** Steven F. Maier, "Behavioral Control Blunts Reactions to Contemporaneous and Future Adverse Events: Medial Prefrontal Cortex Plasticity and a Corticostriatal Network." *Neurobiology of Stress* 1 (2015): 12–22.

131 **This rat doesn't become depressed:** J. Amat et al., "Behavioral Control over Shock Blocks Behavioral and Neurochemical Effects of Later Social Defeat." *Neuroscience* 165, no. 4 (2010): 1031–38.

133 **Researchers who studied the San Pedro Manrique ritual:** Joseph A. Bulbulia et al., "Images from a Jointly-Arousing Collective Ritual Reveal Affective Polarization." *Frontiers in Psychology* 4 (2013): 960.

133 **Humans are not the only species to help:** Erik T. Frank and K. Eduard Linsenmair, "Saving the Injured: Evolution and Mechanisms." *Communicative & Integrative Biology* 10, nos. 5–6 (2017): e1356516; John C. Lilly, "Distress Call of the Bottlenose Dolphin: Stimuli and Evoked Behavioral Responses." *Science* 139, no. 3550 (1963): 116–18; Martijn Hammers and Lyanne Brouwer, "Rescue Behaviour in a Social Bird: Removal of Sticky 'Bird-Catcher Tree' Seeds by Group Members." *Behaviour* 154, no. 4 (2017): 403–11.

134 **philosopher Thomas Brown argued that our muscles:** Thomas Brown, *Lectures on the Philosophy of the Human Mind*, 2nd ed., 4 vols (first published 1820; Edinburgh, 1824). Vol. 1, 460–61. As described in Roger Smith, "'The Sixth Sense': Towards a History of Muscular Sensation." *Gesnerus* 68, no. 2 (2011): 218–71.

135 **The regions of your brain that produce . . . self-awareness:** Olaf Blanke, Mel Slater, and Andrea Serino, "Behavioral, Neural, and Computational Principles of Bodily Self-Consciousness." *Neuron* 88, no. 1 (2015): 145–66.

135 **"My limbs just feel lost":** M. Kelter (a pseudonym used by author), "Descartes' Lantern (the Curious Case of Autism and Proprioception)." August 26, 2014; https://theinvisiblestrings.com/descartes -lantern-curious-case-autism-proprioception/. Quoted with author permission.

137 **"I have seen women who have felt small for years":** Laura Khoudari, "The Incredible, Life-Affirming Nature of the Deadlift." *Medium*, March 1, 2018; https://medium.com/@laura.khoudari/the-incredible -life-affirming-nature-of-the-deadlift-4e1e5b637dad.

144 **"Hope without an object cannot live":** Samuel Taylor Coleridge, quote from the 1825 sonnet "Work Without Hope."

144 **C. R. Snyder, who conducted:** C. Richard Snyder, "Hope Theory: Rainbows in the Mind." *Psychological Inquiry* 13, no. 4 (2002): 249–75.

145 **a hill seems less steep:** Simone Schnall et al., "Social Support and the Perception of Geographical Slant." *Journal of Experimental Social Psychology* 44, no. 5 (2008): 1246–55.

145 **In 2007 . . . a sixty-five-year-old man with Parkinson's disease:** Ilana Schlesinger, Ilana Erikh, and David Yarnitsky, "Paradoxical Kinesia at War." *Movement Disorders* 22, no. 16 (2007): 2394–97, as cited in H. G. Laurie Rauch, Georg Schönbächler, and Timothy D. Noakes, "Neural Correlates of Motor Vigour and Motor Urgency During Exercise." *Sports Medicine* 43, no. 4 (2013): 227–41.

146 **When people who are important to you celebrate:** Harry T. Reis et al., "Are You Happy for Me? How Sharing Positive Events with Others Provides Personal and Interpersonal Benefits." *Journal of Personality and Social Psychology* 99, no. 2 (2010): 311–29.

147 **physician Jerome Groopman defines hope:** Jerome Groopman, *The Anatomy of Hope: How People Prevail in the Face of Illness* (New York: Random House Trade Paperbacks, 2005). Quote appears on p. xiv.

147 **In one experiment, psychologists induced hope:** Carla J. Berg, C. R. Snyder, and Nancy Hamilton, "The Effectiveness of a Hope Intervention in Coping with Cold Pressor Pain." *Journal of Health Psychology* 13, no. 6 (2008): 804–9.

147 **when people perceive a painful physical exercise:** Fabrizio Benedetti et al., "Pain as a Reward: Changing the Meaning of Pain from Negative to Positive Co-activates Opioid and Cannabinoid Systems." *PAIN* 154, no. 3 (2013): 361–67.

148 **"When I watch Kobe glide to the basket":** Jonah Lehrer, "The Neuroscience of Fandom." *Frontal Cortex,* June 13, 2008; http://scienceblogs.com/cortex/2008/06/13/it-happens-to-me-every/.

149 **"When we see a human body moving:** "John Joseph Martin, *America Dancing: The Background and Personalities of the Modern Dance* (1936; reprint, Brooklyn, NY: Dance Horizons, 1968). Quote appears on p. 117.

Chapter 6: Embrace Life

155 **Psychologists call physical activity:** For an excellent introduction to green exercise, see: Jo Barton, Rachel Bragg, Carly Wood, and Jules Pretty, eds., *Green Exercise: Linking Nature, Health and Well-Being* (New York: Routledge, 2016).

155 **Taking a walk outdoors slows:** Mariya Davydenko and Johanna Peetz, "Time Grows on Trees: The Effect of Nature Settings on Time Perception." *Journal of Environmental Psychology* 54 (2017): 20–26.

155 **Simply being in an environment:** Richard A. Fuller et al., "Psychological Benefits of Greenspace Increase with Biodiversity." *Biology Letters* 3, no. 4 (2007): 390–94.

155 **Even just remembering a time:** Michelle N. Shiota, Dacher Keltner, and Amanda Mossman, "The Nature of Awe: Elicitors, Appraisals, and Effects on Self-Concept." *Cognition and Emotion* 21, no. 5 (2007): 944–63.

156 **"There were no sharp things inside me":** Paul Heintzman, "Men's Wilderness Experience and Spirituality: A Qualitative Study." *Proceedings of the 2006 Northeastern Recreation Research Symposium,* General Technical Report NRS-P-14, 216–25; https://www.nrs.fs.fed.us/pubs/gtr/gtr_nrs-p-14/30-heintzman-p-14.pdf.

156 **"a complete sense of belonging":** Robert D. Schweitzer, Harriet L. Glab, and Eric Brymer, "The Human–Nature Experience: A Phenomenological-Psychoanalytic Perspective." *Frontiers in Psychology* 9 (2018): 969; https://doi.org/10.3389/fpsyg.2018.00969.

156 **At the Hong-reung Arboretum:** Won Kim et al., "The Effect of Cognitive Behavior Therapy-Based Psychotherapy Applied in a Forest Environment on Physiological Changes and Remission of Major Depressive Disorder." *Psychiatry Investigation* 6, no. 4 (2009): 245–54.

156 **In an Austrian study, adding mountain hiking:** J. Sturm, "Physical Exercise Through Mountain Hiking in High-Risk Suicide Patients. A Randomized Crossover Trial." *Acta Psychiatrica Scandinavica* 126, no. 6 (2012): 467–75.

157 **"I felt more free, less trapped":** Maura Kelly, "Finally Seeing the Forest for the Trees." Longreads, November 2017; https://longreads.com/2017/11/15/finally-seeing-the-forest-for-the-trees/. Some quotes and details come from a series of email interviews I conducted with Kelly.

158 **This brain network was first identified:** Marcus E. Raichle et al., "A Default Mode of Brain Function." *Proceedings of the National Academy of Sciences of the USA* 98, no. 2 (2001): 676–82.

158–59 **The brain's baseline activity:** Christopher G. Davey and Ben J. Harrison, "The Brain's Center of Gravity: How the Default Mode Network Helps Us to Understand the Self." *World Psychiatry* 17, no. 3 (2018): 278–79.

159 **However, the default state also has a downside:** Igor Marchetti et al., "Spontaneous Thought and Vulnerability to Mood Disorders: The Dark Side of the Wandering Mind." *Clinical Psychological Science* 4, no. 5 (2016): 835–57.

159 **people who suffer from depression or anxiety:** Aneta Brzezicka, "Integrative Deficits in Depression and in Negative Mood States as a Result of Fronto-Parietal Network Dysfunctions." *Acta Neurobiol Exp* 73, no. 3 (2013): 313–25; Igor Marchetti et al., "The Default Mode Network and Recurrent Depression: A Neurobiological Model of Cognitive Risk Factors." *Neuropsychology Review* 22, no. 3 (2012): 229–51; Annette Beatrix Brühl et al., "Neuroimaging in Social Anxiety Disorder—A Meta-Analytic Review Resulting in a New Neurofunctional Model." *Neuroscience & Biobehavioral Reviews* 47 (2014): 260–80; Claudio Gentili et al., "Beyond Amygdala: Default Mode Network Activity Differs Between Patients with Social Phobia and Healthy Controls." *Brain Research Bulletin* 79, no. 6 (2009): 409–13.

159 **The brain's reward system . . . can become highly connected:** Li Wang et al., "Altered Default Mode and Sensorimotor Network Connectivity with Striatal Subregions in Primary Insomnia: A Resting-State Multi-Band fMRI Study." *Frontiers in Neuroscience* 12 (2018): 917; doi: 10.3389/fnins.2018.00917.

159–60 **In brain-imaging studies, focused breathing, mindfulness, and repeating a mantra:** Kathleen A. Garrison et al., "Meditation Leads to Reduced Default Mode Network Activity Beyond an Active Task." *Cognitive, Affective, & Behavioral Neuroscience* 15, no. 3 (2015): 712–20; Judson A. Brewer et al., "Meditation Experience Is Associated with Differences in Default Mode Network Activity and Connectivity." *Proceedings of the National Academy of Sciences of the USA* 108, no. 50 (2011): 20254–59; Rozalyn Simon et al., "Mantra Meditation Suppression of Default Mode Beyond an Active Task: A Pilot Study." *Journal of Cognitive Enhancement* 1, no. 2 (2017): 219–27.

160 **In one unusual case study:** Yochai Ataria, Yair Dor-Ziderman, and Aviva Berkovich-Ohana, "How Does It Feel to Lack a Sense of Boundaries? A Case Study of a Long-Term Mindfulness Meditator." *Consciousness and Cognition* 37 (2015): 133–47; Yair Dor-Ziderman et al., "Mindfulness-Induced Selflessness: A MEG Neurophenomenological Study." *Frontiers in Human Neuroscience* 7 (2013): 582.

160 **At least one study has tried to capture this effect:** Gregory N. Bratman et al., "Nature Experience Reduces Rumination and Subgenual Prefrontal Cortex Activation." *Proceedings of the National Academy of Sciences of the USA* 112, no. 28 (2015): 8567–72.

160 **Individuals who suffer from depression show:** J. Paul Hamilton et al., "Depressive Rumination, the Default-Mode Network, and the Dark Matter of Clinical Neuroscience." *Biological Psychiatry* 78, no. 4 (2015): 224–30.

161 **Magnetically stimulating the prefrontal cortex:** Conor Liston et al., "Default Mode Network Mechanisms of Transcranial Magnetic Stimulation in Depression." *Biological Psychiatry* 76, no. 7 (2014): 517–26.

161 **Intravenous infusions of the drug ketamine:** Milan Scheidegger et al., "Ketamine Decreases Resting State Functional Network Connectivity in Healthy Subjects: Implications for Antidepressant Drug Action." *PLOS ONE* 7, no. 9 (2012): e44799.

161 **This may explain why the psychological benefits:** Femke Beute and Yvonne A. W. de Kort, "The Natural Context of Wellbeing: Ecological Momentary Assessment of the Influence of Nature and Daylight on Affect and Stress for Individuals with Depression Levels Varying from None to Clinical." *Health & Place* 49 (2018): 7–18.

161 **"Diving into wild water is the great bringer-back of reality":** Andrew Fusek Peters, *Dip: Wild Swims from the Borderlands* (London: Rider, 2014). Quotes appear on pp. 143 and 212.

162 **the default mode is relentlessly verbal:** Elena Makovac et al., "The Verbal Nature of Worry in Generalized Anxiety: Insights from the Brain." *NeuroImage: Clinical* 17 (2017): 882–92.

162 **Mindfulness practices teach people:** Norman A. S. Farb et al., "Attending to the Present: Mindfulness Meditation Reveals Distinct Neural Modes of Self-Reference." *Social Cognitive and Affective Neuroscience* 2, no. 4 (2007): 313–22.

162 **Among highly experienced meditators:** Veronique A. Taylor et al. "Impact of Meditation Training on the Default Mode Network During a Restful State." *Social Cognitive and Affective Neuroscience* 8, no. 1 (2013): 4–14; Richard Harrison et al., "Trait Mindfulness Is Associated with Lower Pain Reactivity and Connectivity of the Default Mode Network." *Journal of Pain* (2018); https://doi.org/10.1016/j.jpain.2018.10.011.

163 **two pressures shaped the development of the human brain:** Alexandra G. Rosati, "Foraging Cognition: Reviving the Ecological Intelligence Hypothesis." *Trends in Cognitive Sciences* 21, no. 9 (2017): 691–702.

165 **Like green exercise, these drugs alter consciousness:** Fernanda Palhano-Fontes et al., "The Psychedelic State Induced by Ayahuasca Modulates the Activity and Connectivity of the Default Mode Network." *PLOS ONE* 10, no. 2 (2015): e0118143; Robin L. Carhart-Harris et al., "Neural Correlates of the Psychedelic State as Determined by fMRI Studies with Psilocybin." *Proceedings of the National Academy of Sciences of the USA* 109, no. 6 (2012): 2138–43.

165 **During an LSD trip:** Enzo Tagliazucchi et al., "Increased Global Functional Connectivity Correlates with LSD-Induced Ego Dissolution." *Current Biology* 26, no. 8 (2016): 1043–50.

165 **intense spiritual experience while in nature:** Terry Louise Terhaar, "Evolutionary Advantages of Intense Spiritual Experience in Nature." *Journal for the Study of Religion, Nature & Culture* 3, no. 3 (2009): 303–39.

165 **"I didn't just feel amazing. I felt free":** Rich Roll, *Finding Ultra: Rejecting Middle Age, Becoming One of the World's Fittest Men, and Discovering Myself* (New York: Crown/Three Rivers Press, 2012). Quote appears on p. 13.

165–66 **"I felt a complete merging":** Woman's hiking anecdote and quote appears in Laura M. Fredrickson and Dorothy H. Anderson, "A Qualitative Exploration of the Wilderness Experience as a Source of Spiritual Inspiration." *Journal of Environmental Psychology* 19, no. 1 (1999): 21–39.

166 **Analyses of journal entries:** Kathryn E. Schertz et al., "A Thought in the Park: The Influence of Naturalness and Low-Level Visual Features on Expressed Thoughts." *Cognition* 174 (2018): 82–93.

167 **"Connecting with nature embeds us more deeply":** Holli-Anne Passmore and Andrew J. Howell, "Eco-Existential Positive Psychology: Experiences in Nature, Existential Anxieties, and Well-Being." *The Humanistic Psychologist* 42, no. 4 (2014): 370–88.

167 **walking in a nature reserve for fifteen minutes:** F. Stephan Mayer et al., "Why Is Nature Beneficial? The Role of Connectedness to Nature." *Environment and Behavior* 41, no. 5 (2009): 607–43.

168 **In 2013, the city of Melbourne, Australia:** You can explore the map of Melbourne's trees and email a tree here: http://melbourneurbanforestvisual.com.au/#mapexplore.

169 **The human longing to connect with nature:** Stephen R. Kellert and Edward O. Wilson, eds., *The Biophilia Hypothesis* (Washington, DC: Island Press, 1993).

169 **individuals who feel a stronger connection to nature:** Colin A. Capaldi, Raelyne L. Dopko, and John M. Zelenski, "The Relationship Between Nature Connectedness and Happiness: A Meta-Analysis." *Frontiers in Psychology* 5 (2014): doi: 10.3389/fpsyg.2014.00976; Anne Cleary et al., "Exploring Potential Mechanisms Involved in the Relationship Between Eudaimonic Wellbeing and Nature Connection." *Landscape and Urban Planning* 158 (2017): 119–28.

169 **People who make more frequent visits to natural spaces:** M. P. White et al., "Natural Environments and Subjective Wellbeing: Different Types of Exposure Are Associated with Different Aspects of Wellbeing." *Health & Place* 45 (2017): 77–84.

169 **One study tracked the daily movements:** George MacKerron and Susana Mourato, "Happiness Is Greater in Natural Environments." *Global Environmental Change* 23, no. 5 (2013): 992–1000.

169 **Americans spend 93 percent of their time indoors:** Neil E. Klepeis et al., "The National Human Activity Pattern Survey (NHAPS): A Resource for Assessing Exposure to Environmental Pollutants." *Journal of Exposure Analysis and Environmental Epidemiology* 11, no. 3 (2001): 231–52.

170 **Many listen to recordings:** I learned this fact from Scott Kelly, *Endurance: My Year in Space, A Lifetime of Discovery* (New York: Knopf, 2017).

170 **On one expedition, American astronaut and flight engineer Don Pettit:** Details about Pettit's space station garden are drawn from multiple reports and previously published interviews, including his NASA chronicles and Letters from Space blog (https://blogs.nasa.gov /letters/author/dpettitblog/; and https://spaceflight.nasa.gov/station /crew/exp6/spacechronicles.html) as well as Debbora Battaglia, "Aeroponic Gardens and Their Magic: Plants/Persons/Ethics in Suspension." *History and Anthropology* 28, no. 3 (2017): 263–92.

171 **"When we relate to nature":** Rollo May, *Man's Search for Himself* (New York: Norton, 2009). Quote appears on p. 49.

171 **the *old friends hypothesis*:** Christopher A. Lowry et al., "The Microbiota, Immunoregulation, and Mental Health: Implications for Public Health." *Current Environmental Health Reports* 3, no. 3 (2016): 270–86.

171 **the lack of exposure to dirt in modern society:** Graham A. W. Rook, Charles L. Raison, and Christopher A. Lowry, "Childhood Microbial Experience, Immunoregulation, Inflammation, and Adult Susceptibility to Psychosocial Stressors and Depression." In Bernhard T. Baune, ed., *Inflammation and Immunity in Depression: Basic Science and Clinical Applications* (Cambridge, MA: Academic Press, 2018), 17–44; Charles L. Raison, Christopher A. Lowry, and Graham A. W. Rook,

"Inflammation, Sanitation, and Consternation: Loss of Contact with Coevolved, Tolerogenic Microorganisms and the Pathophysiology and Treatment of Major Depression." *Archives of General Psychiatry* 67, no. 12 (2010): 1211–24.

173 **"You can just be yourself":** Quote from public tweet shared by the Conservation Volunteers Hollybush on October 15, 2018.

173 **women with breast cancer reported . . . a "shoulder-to-shoulder support":** Aileen V. Ireland et al., "Walking Groups for Women with Breast Cancer: Mobilising Therapeutic Assemblages of Walk, Talk and Place." *Social Science & Medicine* (2018): https://doi.org/10.1016 /j.socscimed.2018.03.016.

174 **A 2017 analysis of urban community gardens:** Søren Christensen, "Seeding Social Capital? Urban Community Gardening and Social Capital." *Civil Engineering and Architecture* 5, no. 3 (2017): 104–23.

174 **"Whereas before it was just my home":** J. Mailhot, "Green Social Work and Community Gardens: A Case Study of the North Central Community Gardens." Master's thesis, University of Nordland, Bodo, Norway, 2015.

174–75 **The Beach 91st Street Community Garden:** Joana Chan, Bryce DuBois, and Keith G. Tidball, "Refuges of Local Resilience: Community Gardens in Post-Sandy New York City." *Urban Forestry & Urban Greening* 14, no. 3 (2015): 625–35. Quote appears on p. 631.

175 **"People must belong to a tribe":** E. O. Wilson, *Consilience: The Unity of Knowledge* (New York: Knopf, 1998). Quote appears on p. 6.

175 **volunteers reported an increase in optimism:** 2016 National Evaluation of Green Gym, supported by the New Economics Foundation (NEF). Full report available at https://www.tcv.org.uk/sites/default/files/green-gym -evaluation-report-2016.pdf.

176 **In 2017, researchers at the University of Westminster:** This study has not yet been published in a scientific journal, but you can learn more about it at https://www.tcv.org.uk/greengym/trust-me-im-a-doctor/university -westminster-findings.

176–77 **In cities as diverse as Delhi, London, and Milwaukee:** Debarati Mukherjee et al., "Park Availability and Major Depression in Individuals with Chronic Conditions: Is There an Association in Urban India?" *Health & Place* 47 (2017): 54–62; Mathew P. White et al., "Would You Be Happier Living in a Greener Urban Area? A Fixed-Effects Analysis of Panel Data." *Psychological Science* 24, no. 6 (2013): 920–28; Kirsten M. M. Beyer et al., "Exposure to Neighborhood Green Space and Mental Health: Evidence from the Survey of the Health of Wisconsin." *International Journal of Environmental Research and Public Health* 11, no. 3 (2014): 3453–72.

177 **When the Pennsylvania Horticultural Society:** Eugenia C. South et al., "Effect of Greening Vacant Land on Mental Health of Community-Dwelling

Adults: A Cluster Randomized Trial." *JAMA Network Open* 1, no. 3 (2018): e180298.

177–78 **"Root growth is essentially opportunistic":** Thomas O. Perry, "Tree Roots: Facts and Fallacies." *Arnoldia* 49, no. 4 (1989): 3–24.

Chapter 7: How We Endure

181 **In North America alone:** Statistics about ultramarathon participation in North America are from http://realendurance.com/summary.php.

181 **"reminds us that through adversity there is hope":** Comrades Marathon, "Beginnings"; http://www.comrades.com/marathoncentre /club-details/8-news/latest-news/326-history-of-comrades.

181 **the word *athlete* derives from:** Robin Harvie, *The Lure of Long Distances: Why We Run* (New York: Public Affairs, 2011). Quote appears on p. 140.

185 **"the passage of time turned into a dragging":** David Heinz, Victor Vogel, et al., "Disturbed Experience of Time in Depression-Evidence from Content Analysis." *Frontiers in Human Neuroscience* 12 (2018): 66.

185 **runners reported "distortions in time":** Dolores A. Christensen, "Over the Mountains and Through the Woods: Psychological Processes of Ultramarathon Runners." PhD dissertation, Springfield College, 2017.

185 **Ultrarunner Robin Harvie remembers reaching:** Harvie, *The Lure of Long Distances*. Quotes appear on pp. 239–40 and 67.

185 **"You don't have to get rid of the pain":** Jennifer Pharr Davis, *The Pursuit of Endurance: Harnessing the Record-Breaking Power of Strength and Resilience* (New York: Viking, 2018). Quote appears on p. 293.

185–86 **Researcher Karen Weekes followed ten athletes:** Karen Weekes, "Cognitive Coping Strategies and Motivational Profiles of Ultra-Endurance Athletes." PhD dissertation, Dublin City University, 2004.

188 **"a series of brutal, soul-crushing hills":** Torres shared this story in our conversation; some details and quotes also are drawn from her essay about the Kauai Marathon experience at https://christinatorres .org/2016/09/21/the-sweetness-of-surrender-kauai-marathon-2016/.

190 **"being alive is more important than hands and feet":** "Yukon Arctic Ultra Racer May Lose Hands, Feet to Frostbite." CBC News, February 14, 2018; http://www.cbc.ca/news/canada/north/yukon-arctic-ultra -zanda-pollhammer-1.4535514.

190 **Kirsty-Ann Burroughs interviewed endurance runners:** Kirsty-Ann Burroughs, "Faith and Endurance: The Relationship Between Distinct Theologies and the Experience of Running for Christian Women." PhD dissertation, University of Brighton, 2004.

191 **researchers analyzed the hormones:** Robert H. Coker et al., "Metabolic Responses to the Yukon Arctic Ultra: Longest and Coldest in the

World." *Medicine and Science in Sports and Exercise* 49, no. 2 (2017): 357–62.

191 **irisin also has powerful effects on the brain:** Christiane D. Wrann et al., "Exercise Induces Hippocampal BDNF Through a PGC-1α/ FNDC5 Pathway." *Cell Metabolism* 18, no. 5 (2013): 649–59; David A. Raichlen and Gene E. Alexander, "Adaptive Capacity: An Evolutionary Neuroscience Model Linking Exercise, Cognition, and Brain Health." *Trends in Neurosciences* 40, no. 7 (2017): 408–21; Ning Chen et al., "Irisin, an Exercise-Induced Myokine as a Metabolic Regulator: An Updated Narrative Review." *Diabetes/Metabolism Research and Reviews* 32, no. 1 (2016): 51–59.

191 **Lower levels are associated with an increased risk of depression:** Wen-Jun Tu et al., "Decreased Level of Irisin, a Skeletal Muscle Cell-Derived Myokine, Is Associated with Post-Stroke Depression in the Ischemic Stroke Population." *Journal of Neuroinflammation* 15, no. 1 (2018): 133; Csaba Papp et al., "Alteration of the Irisin-Brain-Derived Neurotrophic Factor Axis Contributes to Disturbance of Mood in COPD Patients." *International Journal of Chronic Obstructive Pulmonary Disease* 12 (2017): 2023–33.

191 **elevated levels can boost motivation:** Judit Zsuga et al., "FNDC5/ Irisin, a Molecular Target for Boosting Reward-Related Learning and Motivation." *Medical Hypotheses* 90 (2016): 23–28.

191 **Injecting the protein directly into the brains of mice:** Aline Siteneski et al., "Central Irisin Administration Affords Antidepressant-Like Effect and Modulates Neuroplasticity-Related Genes in the Hippocampus and Prefrontal Cortex of Mice." *Progress in Neuro-Psychopharmacology and Biological Psychiatry* 84 (2018): 294–303.

191 **Higher blood levels of irisin:** Muaz Belviranli et al., "The Relationship Between Brain-Derived Neurotrophic Factor, Irisin and Cognitive Skills of Endurance Athletes." *Physician and Sportsmedicine* 44, no. 3 (2016): 290–96; Yunho Jin et al., "Molecular and Functional Interaction of the Myokine Irisin with Physical Exercise and Alzheimer's Disease." *Molecules* 23, no. 12 (2018): e3229; Dong-Jie Li et al., "The Novel Exercise-Induced Hormone Irisin Protects Against Neuronal Injury via Activation of the Akt and ERK½ Signaling Pathways and Contributes to the Neuroprotection of Physical Exercise in Cerebral Ischemia." *Metabolism* 68 (2017): 31–42.

191–92 **Irisin . . . is the best-known example of a *myokine*:** Ning Chen et al., "Irisin, an Exercise-Induced Myokine as a Metabolic Regulator: An Updated Narrative Review." *Diabetes/Metabolism Research and Reviews* 32, no. 1 (2016): 51–59.

192 **One of the greatest recent scientific breakthroughs:** For an introduction to the concept of myokines, see: Martin Whitham and

Mark A. Febbraio, "The Ever-Expanding Myokinome: Discovery Challenges and Therapeutic Implications." *Nature Reviews Drug Discovery* 15, no. 10 (2016): 719–29; Svenia Schnyder and Christoph Handschin, "Skeletal Muscle as an Endocrine Organ: PGC-1α, Myokines and Exercise." *Bone* 80 (2015): 115–25; Jun Seok Son et al., "Exercise-Induced Myokines: A Brief Review of Controversial Issues of This Decade." *Expert Review of Endocrinology & Metabolism* 13, no. 1 (2018): 51–58.

192 **One of these proteins is irisin:** Jill Fox et al., "Effect of an Acute Exercise Bout on Immediate Post-Exercise Irisin Concentration in Adults: A Meta-Analysis." *Scandinavian Journal of Medicine and Science in Sports* 28, no. 1 (2018): 16–28.

192 **Following a single treadmill workout:** Stella S. Daskalopoulou et al., "Plasma Irisin Levels Progressively Increase in Response to Increasing Exercise Workloads in Young, Healthy, Active Subjects." *European Journal of Endocrinology* 171, no. 3 (2014): 343–52.

192 **A 2018 scientific paper identified thirty-five proteins:** Martin Whitham et al., "Extracellular Vesicles Provide a Means for Tissue Crosstalk During Exercise." *Cell Metabolism* 27, no. 1 (2018): 237–51.

193 **Some myokines even metabolize a neurotoxic chemical:** Leandro Z. Agudelo et al., "Skeletal Muscle PGC-1α1 Modulates Kynurenine Metabolism and Mediates Resilience to Stress-Induced Depression." *Cell* 159, no. 1 (2014): 33–45; Maja Schlittler et al., "Endurance Exercise Increases Skeletal Muscle Kynurenine Aminotransferases and Plasma Kynurenic Acid in Humans." *American Journal of Physiology—Cell Physiology* 310, no. 10 (2016): C836–40.

193 **"hope molecules":** Cristy Phillips and Ahmad Salehi, "A Special Regenerative Rehabilitation and Genomics Letter: Is There a 'Hope' Molecule?" *Physical Therapy* 96, no. 4 (2016): 581–83.

194 **Endurance activities like walking, hiking, jogging:** Brittany A. Edgett et al., "Dissociation of Increases in PGC-1α and Its Regulators from Exercise Intensity and Muscle Activation Following Acute Exercise." *PLOS ONE* 8, no. 8 (2013): e71623; Lee T. Ferris, James S. Williams, and Chwan-Li Shen, "The Effect of Acute Exercise on Serum Brain-Derived Neurotrophic Factor Levels and Cognitive Function." *Medicine & Science in Sports & Exercise* 39, no. 4 (2007): 728–34; Malcolm Eaton et al., "Impact of a Single Bout of High-Intensity Interval Exercise and Short-Term Interval Training on Interleukin-6, FNDC5, and METRNL mRNA Expression in Human Skeletal Muscle." *Journal of Sport and Health Science* 7, no. 2 (2018): 191–96; Ayhan Korkmaz et al., "Plasma Irisin Is Increased Following 12 Weeks of Nordic Walking and Associates with Glucose Homoeostasis in Overweight/Obese Men with Impaired Glucose Regulation." *European Journal of Sport Science* 19, no. 2 (2019): 258–66;

Katya Vargas-Ortiz et al., "Aerobic Training But No Resistance Training Increases SIRT3 in Skeletal Muscle of Sedentary Obese Male Adolescents." *European Journal of Sport Science* 18, no. 2 (2018): 226–34.

194 **Among those who are already active:** Cesare Granata, Nicholas A. Jamnick, and David J. Bishop, "Principles of Exercise Prescription, and How They Influence Exercise-Induced Changes of Transcription Factors and Other Regulators of Mitochondrial Biogenesis." *Sports Medicine* 48, no. 7 (2018): 1541–59; Casper Skovgaard et al., "Combined Speed Endurance and Endurance Exercise Amplify the Exercise-Induced PGC-1α and PDK4 mRNA Response in Trained Human Muscle." *Physiological Reports* 4, no. 14 (2016): e12864.

194 **In one study, running to exhaustion:** Shanhu Qiu et al., "Acute Exercise-Induced Irisin Release in Healthy Adults: Associations with Training Status and Exercise Mode." *European Journal of Sport Science* 18, no. 9 (2018): 1226–33.

197 **"Can there be a better way to work out who you are?":** Quote from Jethro De Decker's personal blog post describing his experience in the 2018 Yukon Arctic Ultra, March 9, 2018; https://nextbigadventure .wordpress.com/2018/03/09/yukon-arctic-ultra-2018/.

198 **In her memoir, *Dirty Inspirations*, she recalls considering her options:** Terri Schneider, *Dirty Inspirations: Lessons from the Trenches of Extreme Endurance Sports* (Hobart, NY: Hatherleigh, 2016). Many of the details about Schneider's adventures come from this memoir; others are from direct conversation, as noted in the text.

203 **After the event, a Canadian competitor:** "50 Stunning Olympic Moments No. 3: Derek Redmond and Dad Finish 400m." *The Guardian*, November 30, 2011; https://www.theguardian.com/sport/blog/2011 /nov/30/50-stunning-olympic-moments-derek-redmond.

204 **"Things seem easier when they're shared":** Quote from participant in Christensen, "Over the Mountains and Through the Woods."

204 **"He gave me his water and walked with me":** Joy Ebertz, "Running Is a Community Sport." *Medium*, April 27, 2017; https://medium.com /@jkebertz/running-is-a-community-sport-ba27dd7a0fb0.

204 **During one ultrarunner's first overnight 62-mile trail race:** Quote from participant in Christensen, "Over the Mountains and Through the Woods."

204 **As one runner explains, "If you have socks":** Jenna M. Quicke, "The Phenomenon of Community: A Qualitative Study of the Ultrarunning Community." PhD dissertation, Prescott College, 2017.

204 **When researcher Jenna Quicke asked ultrarunners to choose a photo:** Quicke, "The Phenomenon of Community."

205 **Sharing a physically painful experience:** Brock Bastian, Jolanda Jetten, and Laura J. Ferris, "Pain as Social Glue: Shared Pain Increases Cooperation." *Psychological Science* 25, no. 11 (2014): 2079–85.

205 **collective rituals that include pain bond us to others:** Harvey Whitehouse and Jonathan A. Lanman, "The Ties That Bind Us: Ritual, Fusion, and Identification." *Current Anthropology* 55, no. 6 (2014): 674–95.

205 **"When you go up there, everyone is your brother":** Dimitris Xygalatas, "The Biosocial Basis of Collective Effervescence: An Experimental Anthropological Study of a Fire-Walking Ritual." *Fieldwork in Religion* 9, no. 1 (2014): 53–67.

206 **According to a survey of hospice care nurses:** Stacey Burling, "What Do Dying People Really Talk About at the End of Life?" *Philadelphia Inquirer*, December 13, 2018; http://www.philly.com/health/what-do -hospice-patients-talk-about-towson-death-regret-family-gratitude -20181214.html.

206 **The Marathon Monks of Mount Hiei, Japan:** John Stevens and Tadashi Namba, *The Marathon Monks of Mount Hiei* (Brattleboro, VT: Echo Point Books & Media, 2013).

206–7 **In 2010, he spoke with National Public Radio:** "Monk's Enlightenment Begins with a Marathon Walk." *Morning Edition*, National Public Radio. May 11, 2010; https://www.npr.org/templates/story/story.php?storyId= 125223168.

Final Thoughts

212 **Norwegian ethicist Sigmund Loland posed the question:** Sigmund Loland, "The Exercise Pill: Should We Replace Exercise with Pharmaceutical Means?" *Sport, Ethics and Philosophy* 11, no. 1 (2017): 63–74.

214 **"the possibilities—the transformative traits of movement":** Doug Anderson, "Recovering Humanity: Movement, Sport, and Nature." *Journal of the Philosophy of Sport* 28, no. 2 (2001): 140–50.

215 **"I was reminded that I wasn't alone":** Quote from dance class participant's email, used with permission.

INDEX

Also by Kelly McGonigal, PhD

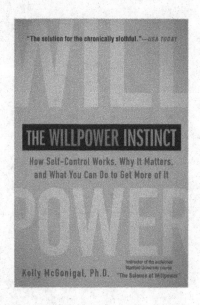

The first book to explain the science of self-control and how it can be harnessed to improve our health, happiness, and productivity.

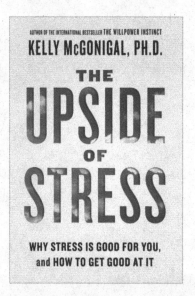

A surprising new view of stress and how to capitalize on its benefits.

AVERY